WEIGHT LOSS & MUSCLE STRENGTH

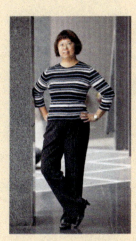
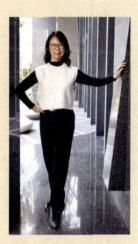

Comfort Zone Strategy towards Freedom

Dr. I Han 韓宜 博士

WEIGHT LOSS & MUSCLE STRENGTH:

Comfort Zone Strategy towards Freedom

Dr. I Han

PhD of International Business, National Taiwan University/ Taipei

Associate Professor of International Business, Feng Chia University/ Taichung

Founder of Agra Boutique Social Enterprise/ Taiwan

Director of Formosan Farms Limited/ England & Wales

To Paul Sherring

I know nothing, but I know people.

I am not a medical doctor, but I feel what makes me better.

I studied social and natural sciences, but I realise the universe tells much more.

I am not superstitious, but I believe in life journeys.

Contents

Foreword

Acknowledgement

Preface

Chapter 1. Academic Career & Social Entrepreneurship

Chapter 2. What University Never Taught

Chapter 3. What Asian Value Never Appreciates

Chapter 4. Food & Weight Loss

Chapter 5. Chinese Medical Training: A Holistic View

Chapter 6. Pai Da Gong: The Easiest Exercise

Chapter 7. Weight Training: The Muscle Strength

Chapter 8. Implications & Get Started

Chapter 9. Qi-Gong Healer, Quantum, and Beyond

References

Foreword

As soon as I was invited to review this book recommended by Charlotte Palmer and Paul Sherring, I knew it would be good and I was not disappointed.

Diet, nutrition and exercise are the possible biggest bones of contention these days. The misinformation is astonishing.

Dr Han pops the bubble of nonsense around nutrition and homes straight into the bullseye which can be summarised as:
Work with your body, not against it;
Let your body work in the way it was designed;
if you eat things your body can't tolerate, you will not be healthy.

It's that simple. Then she explains how to do this.

Simply, the correct input of food in accordance with what suits you, the correct output of exercise in accordance with what you can do.

I like this ultra simple explanation of what can be very confusing and difficult.

Anyone looking for manageable solutions to weight issues will love this.

Sue Cook

BSc (Hons) Lic LCCH.

January 2024/ England

Author of *Nutrition for Special Needs: What shall I feed my child?: Volume 7 (brainbuzzz)*

Author of *Eat for your brain 2: find the right superfood symptom support*

I have known Dr. Han for many years.

We first met in the national program of talented students in sciences and math in Taiwan. Through the rigorous selection process, we both were admitted with full scholarship to the Physics department of National Taiwan University. It was quite an honour at our young age and created a special bonding between us as in the TV sitcom Friends.

Throughout the years, both Dr. Han and I took a few turns in our lives. Dr. Han shifted her study and career to become a professor in international business. As time went by, she got deeply involved in organic tea and health. At my side, I moved on to get my PhD in electrical engineering from Stanford and MBA from UC Berkeley. While I was pushing my career forward in the high-tech business in Silicon Valley, my father got liver cancer and passed away. I decided to change my focus to medicine and started my journey in Chinese medicine.

Given the broad experience in multiple disciplines, we share a similar holistic view on life and health. Our scientific background helps us to investigate different approaches in a logical and open-minded way. Instead of accepting status quo blindly, we follow the principles of logical empiricism, i.e. observation, hypothesis, and verification, to deepen our understanding on how one can improve life quality.

This book is the outcome of Dr. Han's persistent effort of pursuing a healthy and balanced lifestyle. She shares her knowledge and experience without reservation. I am sure that you will enjoy reading this book and benefit from it. Let's start the new journey together with Dr. Han!

Andy Lee

PhD Stanford University

Founder of youngQi Integrative Medicine

January 2024/ California

Author of *When Ancient Medical Wisdom Meets Modern Scientific Mind*

This is a book about my radical personal health transformation: to share my weight loss journey, building muscle strength, and much more. I am writing this book upon the request of all my friends about how I did it at the age of 50. I have delivered numerous lecturing courses and speeches to share my personal experience on this journey. Now is the time to share my story with more people globally.

Key points to know:
1. **Delicious food/ no hunger:**
   If you want to lose weight, it is not necessary to keep yourself unsatisfied with boring food or in a state of hunger all the time.
2. **Easy exercise/ stay in the comfort zone*:**
   If you want to build muscle strength, it is not necessary to push yourself hard in keeping up with exercise/ training which you don't really enjoy.

It then easily can becomes a happy sustainable lifestyle with longevity.

* Comfort zone definition in this book (hereafter, Comfort Zone):
In this context the comfort zone is not framed negatively: fitness can be gained within your own limits and level of comfort, without stress. I have learned it is a dynamic concept. In the short term, your Comfort Zone moves up and down according to your physical and mental conditions. In the long term, your Comfort Zone evolves and eventually shifts to the next level.

My family knew me as a lazy person and it was a family joke. Just like many people, I would say "I wanted to lose weight" all the time but took no meaningful or effective action.

All of that has now changed. Weight loss is not something that I have to constantly remind myself about.

My weight is now stable regardless of how much delicious food I eat (within my stomach limit).

During my 20s and 30s, I tried numerous methods including hard core exercise, but it did not last long. In fact, anything that is not easy will NOT sustain for long, as it is human nature to not commit to anything challenging for too long.

I am a self confessed lazy person. Historically I have never liked to do any exercise unless I had to achieve something (e.g., cycling around Taiwan). Never did I even enter a gym.

Now I exercise daily, and I attend gym workouts every other day.

Anything that is not interesting will not be pleasurable to me. It is human nature. I believe that there are many reading this with similar thoughts/ experiences. That's the purpose, to share with you my own journey: an easy to do strategy as "happy" solutions in this book.

Find your own Comfort Zone; make progress towards your own health and fitness freedom.

Dr. I Han
February 2024/ England

Acknowledgement

This is not a book to gloat and tell you how good I have been. It is a book that shares with you my journey and what I found effective, potentially making everything easy and achievable if you can find your own path with the ideal experts, and communities that suit you. This book is a personal approach, but you will see the possibility for yourself and your loved ones if you've a lot of questions regarding weight loss/ control and exercise/ muscle strength.

It was all these people who participated in a major part of my journey in the past few years. They guided me to become a new me!

I am grateful to the universe for leading me to this major transformation in my 50s. There are many angels/ gatekeepers who have opened an avenue for me. Here I only list some of them. Forgive me if you are not mentioned here but without you, I would not be here.

- My Qi Gong healer, **Mr. Han-Ching Lin**, who supported my health condition not just physically but also mentally and spiritually since 2015, whenever I am in Taiwan. He made me ready for this journey.

- One year and three months, from December 2019 to February 2021, my journey of weight loss by only FOOD, was contributed by the food specialists, **Paul Sherring** and **Charlotte Palmer**, in England.

- My Pai Da Gong teacher, **Carol Lai**, who let me find an easy exercise which is not hard to do every day.

- **Dr. Wen-yu Li** taught me Auricular treatment and offered me many volunteer tours.

- **Dr. Mingchen Lin** taught me pulse-measure diagnosis, and offered me mentorship at his Chinese clinics to learn and discuss from real cases.

- **Benjamin Pluke**, my Osteopathic doctor in London, always looks after my posture, muscle strength, and much more, from a holistic point of view.

- **Ian Dowe, Mr. Universe/ World Championships**, is the one who contributed the "last mile" of building the muscle strength. He guided and trained me for fitness and strength during April-June 2023 in his Dowe Dynamics Gym in London.

Now I am passing my greatest gratitude to you. Bless you to connect to your gatekeepers and build your own way towards the result you want!

Last but not the least, I am the second generation in Taiwan, with both my parents from mainland China during WWII. I am not a native English writer. I use plain and easy English to share my journey with you. For non-English readers, this book is not very difficult to understand. Also, all the photos in this book are original, which means no editing after the shot. I prefer everything natural, so I keep everything as authentic as it should be.

Enjoy!

Preface

If you are seeking the best solution for weight loss and muscle strength, hear my story. Not one ideal methodology, but there are tailored bespoke programmes for everyone, to seek an ideal fit to serve your purpose.

If you are looking for good advice from mainstream authorities, think again. I've been trained by a social science researcher, so I always ask the question: if the trusted authorities do have the answers and can really deliver effective results why don't they? If this was the case would we be dealing with rising national and global metabolic syndrome?

This is a book to share my personal and extraordinary health journey from 2019 to 2023, which has been a major milestone in my own transformation. If you'd like to be influenced by these valuable lessons, this is a book recommended for you, especially if you've tried numerous other avenues that never worked or never lasted. If you know the importance of food/ diet, but you are still looking for "cheat days", this is a book to open the pathway for plenty of delicious food without even any desire or cheating. It is vital to know how critical exercise is to build muscle strength. We as humans always find an excuse not to exercise. This is a book to inspire you to embrace and establish an exercise routine without pain or resistance.

Who am I?

I was an overweight professor teaching at a university in Taiwan. The stress of meeting deadlines of research, teaching, and publishing was an overwhelming excuse not to exercise or cook at home. In fact, I never cooked at home before the start of this journey in 2019.

I was confident in myself in my intellectual performance, but never wanted to face myself in the mirror. When I was reminded by some close friends, I usually responded:
"I cannot lose weight, besides I don't eat much. Probably I possess the fat gene. I do not have a good body shape probably because I have a good brain. God is fair......"
I seldom wore a dress, probably less than I can count on my ten fingers, because I was not bothered by how people were looking at me. I did not care because I did not know how to care for my body/ shape.

My average shape 2010-2019

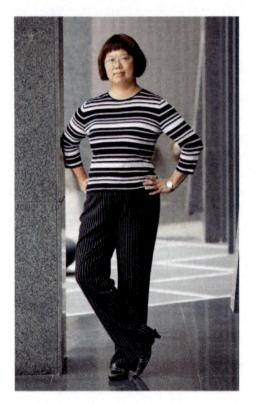

My average shape 2021-2024

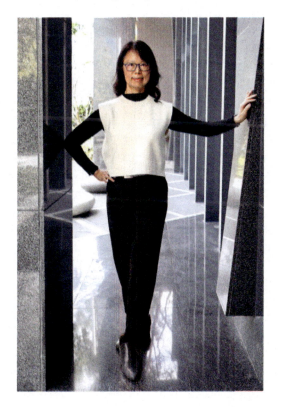

Source: Dr. I Han

It's a long journey to get here.

Initially in the 1990s, I spent a large amount of money on my first weight-loss programme, NTD100,000 (£2,500) for 10kg weight loss with a then famous nutrition-expert company, Jordon Weight-loss Centre (喬登減肥中心) in Taipei when I was 20+ years old. I was joking my meat was worth NTD10,000 (£250) per kilogram!

I was very much an outdoors girl while in college. I was the leader of the Cycling Club at National Taiwan University when I was 19 years old. I went on many cycling trips, including the around-Taiwan-trip. However, I gained 10kg more weight since then, from 58kg to 68kg. I could not understand why my intensive cycling exercise made me a fat girl?!

At Jordon, they asked me to count calories. It was straightforward. As I learned in high school, as more calories are consumed than burned, I put more weight on our body. Over time I successfully lost 10kg by controlling daily consumption of calories: 8-8-2, 8 units carbs, 8 units protein, 2 units fat, with no restriction on vegetables. They showed me how to count those units and requested me to put in their forms as dairy. It was an extremely boring period of eating. Meat was boiled, vegetables were boiled, boiled food without fat was the best idea to keep the dairy, not exceeding the allowed units.

After that, unfortunately, I regained 15kg after a year of Jordon's programme, simply because it was too difficult to sustain, over an extended period of time.

Secondly, I was busy working at FarEasTone Telecom after graduating from my MBA during 1998-2000. Not much time was invested on lunch or dinner. I then decided to cut every meal in half, to save eating time, and to lose weight (according to the previous calories-based Jordon programme). Thanks to burying myself in the busy job, there was no extra time to eat more even when I was hungry. I successfully lost 10kg myself, without spending any money which I was proud of at the time.

But unfortunately, after a year I regained 15kg. I left the busy job at FarEasTone, when I had my son born on the second year of my doctoral programme at National Taiwan University. Since then, I had kept my weight between 75 to 80kg, regardless of whatever weight-loss method I tried.

When I finally met Paul Sherring in London in 2019, I made a fascinating discovery that challenged all of my previous ideas about health and fitness. He roasted a big chicken for me which we shared with his friend Charlotte Palmer at dinner. I was 78kg at that time (not the worst time). He put three pieces of chicken on my plate. I removed the chicken skin completely, as I was taught at Jordon: animal skin contains a lot of fat. Both Paul and Charlotte were surprised and took those skins from my plate and ate them. I left one piece of chicken and they ate it too. I was wondering why?! They were quite fit but I was fat. They ate more than me, even with the very fatty skin?

Why????

I returned to Taiwan and started my own experiment. I have been through many competitions of natural science experiments since I was in junior high school. I was selected as the special talent in Physics and started superconductor research in National Tsing Hua University laboratory when I was in senior high school. To do a self-assessment of my own body experiment, it is not difficult to control most variables and observe the relevance of the result. In any case, it would not be a complete disaster because I still had 2kg to gain to my record high, 80kg. As I'd always eaten out since college, I never knew how to cook. Taiwan is famous for so many delicious foods everywhere at reasonable prices. Why should I cook at home? I was an idiot cook but I could put a whole chicken into a pot and boil it as a chicken and soup. In the past, I would take the skin off and skimmed off the fat while the soup cooled down, in order to consuming the least amount of fat. However, during my one-week experiment, I kept all the chicken skin and fat, but I lost almost 5kg! I couldn't believe it.

What was wrong?

This revelation posed the question; why did I follow the Jordan nutritional experts but could not manage my weight in the long term?

Why did I do the opposite of what I knew by following the two food specialists in London and lost my weight easily without boring food?

By further instructions from Paul and Charlotte, I do not count calories. I am very satisfied with what I eat without boredom and hunger. Though I have to cook at home, I don't need three meals or more. I eat whenever I am hungry. Fat is an efficient fuel, so I don't feel hungry that often.

Also, the most wonderful thing is I can have delicious desserts! It is so much easier to lose the weight and maintain it on a long-term basis. I eventually lost almost 20kg in one year and three months (2019/12-2021/2), from 78-80kg to 60-62kg. After that, my weight was easily well maintained, until a further loss after I started weight training with Ian Dowe on April 2023.

Paul Sherring was right. My correct weight should be 56-57kg, given my height at 165cm. It was rude to hear that when I first met him and Charlotte in London. But the fact based on his profession told the truth that anyone would not think it will be possibly even closed by some easy practices within 15 months.

Of course, it is my own personal choice by taking other professional opinions outside from the mainstream. I do know that I was not the only one who got frustrated with why I had tried so hard, based on advice from doctors, nutritionists, and books, newspapers, while nothing worked well or lasted long.

If you have the same problem as I did, this is the book for you. You will then realise how to do your own research and experiment, and then build your own theory and practice.

Just as in the famous Tom Cruise movie, *The Minority Report*.
"Who do you trust?
Trust yourself, and, do your own research and practice.
And, find your own easy/ comfortable way which will sustain for long."

If this book becomes one of your gatekeepers, I will be very happy for you. Please drop me an email if you wish:

dr.i.han.uk@gmail.com

Chapter 1

Academic Career & Social Entrepreneurship

What should I teach?

I taught international business, social innovation & CSR, and many other business subjects during my ten years as a full-time associate professor at Feng Chia University, in Taichung Taiwan. Right next to the University campus is a famous night market, a must-see for most tourists in town. However, the numerous food stands are very competitive, which leaves almost no space for any proper cafeteria on- or off-campus. It was a shame that students and faculties at the University could hardly find any healthy food options during the day.

During the exact ten years of my academic career there, I accumulated more weight than I'd like, along with many of my colleagues. We had so many lunch meetings with meal boxes. Eating unhealthy meal boxes while discussing school matters was not good for our health! In addition, I did not exercise enough, even when I did go swimming for an hour almost every late evening. My sister was teasing me: "swimming, especially as you swim slowly, is not enough for you as a routine exercise given you are overweight!"

In the academic career, professors are very busy at researching, teaching, and servicing. As far as I knew, many professors did not stop their unhealthy lifestyle until they were hit with a serious illness. In the "academic ivory tower", unfortunately, there are many narratives which are structured by the established rules in each research domain (Figure 1.1). Any publications accepted in good academic journals must be built upon the previous research, or literature review if you know how to write a thesis/dissertation. The journal editors and reviewers in the knowledge domain determine whether the research can be published or not. Who are these journal editors and reviewers? Of course they've published a good amount of research in that domain. Sometimes, there are editors and journals who would like to publish something beyond the existing domain, like the "frontier" research, which can be slightly out of the existing domains. For example, you can imagine the blue tower is a natural science domain A, the orange tower is a social science domain B, and the green tower is an applied science domain C.

What is science?

In plain words, if you can repeat the same study by using the same methodology, and get a similar result, it is a science. Knowledge domains of A, B, or C can all be "science", but A might not truly consider B or C as another science, because they don't understand each other. In other words, they are not built in the same ivory tower. Also, consider those unknown domains in yellow colours? They might even be different shapes of buildings you could never have imagined. However, those yellow none-tower shapes are not considered as scientific at all. First of all, we don't even know them. Secondly, even if someone knew any of them, nobody has found a methodology to repeat the study.

Thirdly, any research paper is not able to be published because nobody can properly review it. In the academic world, the publication/ revision process upon reviewer/ editor decisions pre-sets the impossibility of any possibility beyond those ivy towers.

So, as described in Rupert Sheldrake's book *The Science Delusion*, they are not considered as science in the academic world, even if they exist or even that important to the human world.

Figure 1.1
Academic World of Narratives

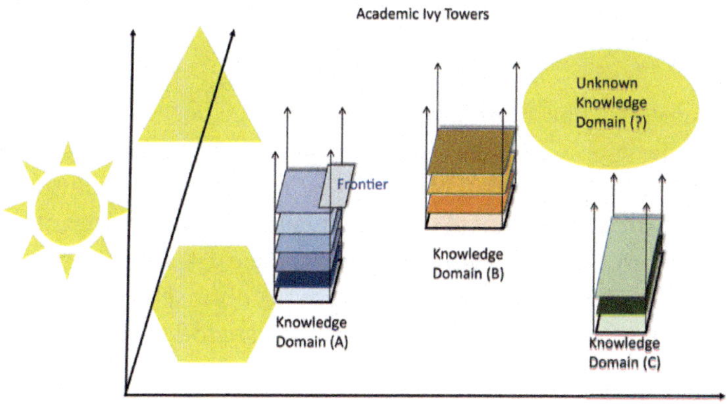

Source: Dr. I Han

My domain used to be social science, or more specifically, international business, strategic management, and social entrepreneurship. However, I had gone through a very challenging publication process when submitting to academic journals because I was studying small farms and farmers and their collaborative relationship in the business management domain. I spent more than five years in this field study, talking to farmers and other stakeholders. I considered my theory built upon the field research which was not within any existing domains. Therefore, later on, I chose to publish my own book of my doctoral dissertation on Amazon. Also, I was lucky to get my tenure with a research book published by New York Macmillan in 2016, *Social Innovation and Business in Taiwan* (with Professor S. Hou as co-author). Based on our field study, a "common good" social innovation can establish sustainable business models for the minority interest groups, such as farmers and rural communities. I then started my social entrepreneurship, Agra Boutique Social Enterprise, in order to prove that our theory of "the common good business model" can work in real practice.

Helping small independent tea farmers become my major business goal at Agra Boutique, as well as promoting other boutique handmade products from rural communities in Taiwan. The products facilitate health, but in the meantime, I did not look healthy at all because of my overweight condition. I taught the consumers to choose authentic teas with sustainable farming methods (pesticide-free, herbicide-free, chemical-free, additive-free) to enhance their health. I taught in hundreds of speeches about my mission to preserve traditional farmhouse hand-processed products, as they become rare in the modern industrial world.

But was I healthy?
Not really.

If I teach something to promote the common good theory in sustainability and health, but I do not know how to put it in real practice, what does that mean?

I used to disagree with professors who teach entrepreneurship but never had their own. That was the lesson I realised when I started up my own social entrepreneurship: I was a business school professor, but I found it was a challenge to build a business in the real world.

During my academic career as a professor, I was not only overweight but my medical report had several items in red (meaning abnormal). I was not happy when I delivered a successful speech or campaign, because I only talked without providing proof.

What should I teach and how?

I trained in Harvard Business School case-teaching method, a methodology to teach students. All my classes were delivered from real practice to realise and apply the theory (which is the opposite to the traditional lecture methodology).

So, if I wanted to sell and promote health in my social entrepreneurship, I would have to become healthy myself in real practice and then, find the theory to teach this real practice.

Self-Assessment

1. What is your career goal?

2. What do you want to achieve?

3. What kind of health condition do you want, given you are happy about #1 & #2?

Chapter 2

What University Never Taught

What does University teach?

Current technology advancement causes a lot of what we were taught in the University to become obsolete overnight. Almost every subject the university teaches can be self-learned online. Almost every technique taught in the university can be delivered by a robot or an AI. What the university never teaches, but which we need the most, is the real practice of achieving something fundamental to our quality of life. The importance of fitness and health, and the maintenance of this in the long term; good health is true wealth and arguably more important than anything else.

I've benefited greatly from farmers and agricultural communities from twenty-year of field research. They've been teaching me what university never teaches, that which benefits me the most; the traditional wisdom of health.

What I learned from farmers is the authentic practice of their lifetime experiences. A selection of these lessons taught can be briefly classified in Table 2.1. It is not what they taught, but how their wisdom became my daily life practices with many check points. Currently there are efforts to bring "food and farming education" into schools. However, the easiest way to learn is to go back to the farm. Seeing, experiencing, touching on the farm and talking to the farmers (choosing different ones from time to time) is the best in-depth learning of a farmers' wisdom. A distant cry from farm life, it is modern life that causes most problems to our health.

Academic researchers always need new contributions to past literature, or so called, conventional wisdom. However, how to improve/ maintain health, by contrast, demands more research to look back on old-fashioned lifestyles beyond the current available literature.

Rural farming communities in Taiwan, and in many developing countries, are probably the slowest to uptake modern technology and lifestyle. What they keep the most, however, is the old wisdom for them to survive well under any circumstances. They work under the extremely hot sun, as well as very harsh rain. The "extreme weather", which has now become a common trendy term, is not new to them. While we sit in the office, eat fast industrial food, and frequent the air-conditioned gym, our detachment from mother nature makes us less healthy, less resilient and weaker than farmers.

In Taiwan, the average educational background of farmers is only at the level of primary school graduates. They are not highly educated so they cannot shift to the well-paid jobs in the much more comfortable venues like most middle-class office workers. But, they are much wiser when it comes to food, health, and lifestyle than those who have never been taught in the university. Nor did I or any other professors understand many other aspects as well as they do. For more details on Tea farmers' lessons please refer to the upcoming book *Formosan Tea* written by me.[1]

Table 2.1
Farmers' wisdom

Farm to Table	Health Dimension	Human Impact
Food grown	Soil Rain Sun Landscape Season Plant variety Eco-system	Artificial interferences: Pesticides Herbicides Chemicals Environmental controls
Food processed	Traditional hand-processed Primary process with machine assistance Industrial sophisticated process	Additives Source of other ingredients Time dimension
Food distributed	Farmer Local farmers' market Local market Regional hub National outlet	Package Time dimension Middlemen
Food purchased	Original format Freshness Trustworthiness	Certification labels Commercial brands

Source: Dr. I Han

I've been teaching "Community-Supported Agriculture in Real Practice" courses at General Education for eight years when I was in Feng Chia University. The "classroom" was a selected agricultural community within one-hour travel distance. Each semester the community might be different. I designed the course to let students see, experience, and touch within the agricultural community and then designed real projects according to real needs. The innovative design of this course was inspired by the years spent with farmers and what I learned from them. This course later won the "Highly Recommended Award: Management Education Practice Award 2018/ Experienced Teaching Practitioner Category, British Academy of Management".

Students who participated in this course might start from having no idea about food at all. Most of them had never ever been to a farm. The best blessing they received was the reconnection to the land, farm, farmer, and agricultural community. It transformed the no-brain diet routine into an appreciation for food. They started to understand and practise the major messages delivered:

1. There is no CP-value in the agricultural industry.
   ☐ Every penny counts. If you want to get better quality, you pay a higher price.
   Simply, there is NO free/ cheap lunch.
2. Find your own trustworthy sources.
   ☐ If you can source back to the origin to the farm/ farmer who produced the food/ tea/ ingredient, it does NOT matter whether it is "certified" as organic/ fair trade/ and similar within the current labelling system. The system is established for consumers who cannot see the origin. Also, those labels can be made-up.
3. Almost every farmer claims their products to be "organic".

☐ If you buy directly from farmers, make sure you do not just "listen" to what they say. It's better to "see" the farm*, or alternatively, you see they eat/drink their own products.

My students will benefit from my course for the rest of their lives. I hope through this book I will be able to bridge the gap of what the university cannot provide you: regain your health—weight loss (or manage, if you are within your right weight) and muscle strength.

My aim is to sell and promote health in my social entrepreneurship, the main objective is to start teaching people what universities never teach: embracing the old wisdom connecting to nature, and real practice in modern settings.

Note:
[1]
Formosan Tea as a book explains the easy to practise methodology to distinguish the "safe" farm and the implications to health in one of the chapters.

Self-Assessment

1. Do you see any other benefits from looking for "cheaper" food, in addition to saving you the money?

2. Did you feel any difference between learning in school vs. learning from any other old wisdom? If yes, which one did you remember the longest?

3. Are you willing to prioritise as number one, a good value, ethically produced and authentic food by taking account of all other possible "costs" if you don't?
Examples: taking the time to use washing-up liquids or vinegar ("intended to remove the pesticides/ chemicals), losing more of your body energy (to process/ absorb more unnecessary compounds from the food), your medical condition (as your body strains to release toxins from organs, blood, cells) that can get inflammation issues or cancer, and so on.

Chapter 3

What Asian Value Never Appreciates

What is the definition of a successful life?

In Taiwan/ Asia, a successful life is defined by how much money you earn, the status or title of your job (such as a medical doctor, a lawyer, or an accountant, or a position in a famous corporation). We have a saying, "If you love hard-working you will win (愛拼就會贏)", but this really the case?

Did every hard-working person win?

Even if it speaks some truth, what will the winning person eventually see as a good result in life?

In the Asian world, getting a high mark and out-performing other peers in academic performance has always been the most important goal since we entered the education system. The "programming" of the ultimate "Asian value" is to win!

Academic winning does not mean anything else but just academic performance.

A friend in Beijing was surprised when she overheard a first-time Yoga-class participant in the gym say: "I am sure that I can do Yoga very well because I graduated from the top university. Yoga exercise is just another easy course to learn." My friend could not understand the relevance between Yoga body movement and university course marks at all. Does a smart head lead to a good result for the body?

Unfortunately, many of them prioritise" their career wins with health and a good quality of life, and they ultimately regret such an exchange. There are many examples of highly paid, high-flying engineers in those high-tech factories in Hsin-chu/ Taichung/ Tainan Industrial Parks, who humbly say: "do not envy our money which we exchange for our health." They are burning the candle at both ends, or working toward a so-called "liver explosion (爆肝)" as the Taiwanese saying goes.

Work, work, work until you die.
Save, save, save until you cannot spend.

What result do you actually get?

Unfortunately, a typical so-called "successful" person in Taiwan/ Asia does not really have a life, especially for the middle-aged plus generations.

Relax, enjoy, and experience a good life. This is probably possible nowadays for the younger Asian generations who are starting to explore themselves and other aspects of life. Everything seems to be challenging, including job/ housing markets, even with a master or doctoral degree from the best university.

So, I concluded if I wanted to sell and promote health in my social entrepreneurship, I should start to teach

the Taiwanese/ Asian what they never appreciated in the past: spend more time out of the university, office, and go into nature. Talk more to real people face to face, not online, and inspire excitement which cheers you up with people you know or new connections, in the middle of the countryside.

Self-Assessment

1. Do you remember any happy, relaxing occasions?

2. When was the last holiday time you really enjoyed?

3. Is it possible to find just one day to fully relax in nature without any phone/ computer interrupted? If yes, please find out whether you can possibly get an idea for your next number 1 & number 2 escape in the future.

Chapter 4

Food & Weight Loss

What is the ideal weight?

When I met Mr. Paul Sherring in November 2019 during my four-day business trip in London, I was not happy about his first words to me:
"Your ideal weight should be about 57kg."

What?

To me, it was rude to meet a man and hear the honest truth, because my weight problems had bothered me for decades.

However, I knew he was probably right, as I was 57 kg during 6 years of my junior and senior high schools. It wasn't until I had moved through university that I started to gain more weight, especially after I was the leader of the Cycling Club at National Taiwan University. At that time, I could not figure it out. The turning point of my weight problems, based on my own explanation (yes, there are always tons of explanations for overweight people, which is very normal, including myself), is that I ate too much after cycling. In fact, Mr. Benjamin Pluke, who became my Osteopathic doctor in London since 2020, taught me that over-exercise would create the opposite result because of the stress hormone, Cortisol (see Chapter 7), including the opposite result of weight-loss.

Mr. Paul Sherring and his friend Ms. Charlotte Palmer have been working as food specialists and naturopathic advisors for decades. The first dinner I had with them, I took the chicken skin off completely, as I was taught at Jordon professional weight-loss centre: animal skin contains a lot of fat, which means high calories (Figure 4.1). Both of them were surprised and took those chicken skins and ate them. I did not eat any of the potatoes, because I avoid the carbohydrates in the late evening time, especially the ones on the plate that looked so oily. Paul and Charlotte were quite fit but I felt fat. This was the beginning of my quest to find out "why".

Figure 4.1.
The dinner with Paul & Charlotte:
oily French chicken with fat-roasted potatoes

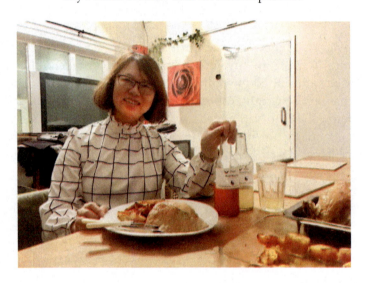

Source: Dr. I Han

I heard so many friends had the similar thoughts as I did:

"Why am I always gaining so much weight even though I've been so careful in eating 'healthy,' keeping calories low?"
" I am hopeless…even if I only drink water, I still gain weight."
" I couldn't give up yummy food just to keep in good shape…otherwise life is too boring."
"I can't be bothered if I have to watch what food to eat all the time in order to keep my weight and shape."
"I will start the weight loss programme tomorrow. This is my last big meal today."
…….

After 15 months of my personal journey, I came to realise that weight loss is not a great mystery. Actually it was easy to lose weight and easy to maintain my "ideal" weight with the right knowledge.

How?

Firstly, what is the "ideal" weight?

It is a simple idea: The structure and content of the body determines weight.

What does that mean?

Imagine a car: If an Audi A3 TSFI car was designed for its structure and the purpose to be driven fast and efficiently, what would be the weight of the car?

What will happen when the five adults are seated in the car with the full trunk of the luggage?

IWhen I did a similar kind of travelling with my family sitting in a full car, I found:
- It was harder to accelerate, so I had to push the gas pedal harder.
- It took a longer distance to stop the car.
- It was less efficient for petrol consumption and less mileage per litre.

So many people asked me how I lost the weight during one year and three months (2019/12-2021/2), from 78-80kg to 60-62kg. It has been just a simple rule:

Eat the "right" food which your body is able to recognise/ digest/ absorb/ dispose of!

It doesn't really matter how much the food is counted by calories. The calories in the food do not translate into a fully burned condition, especially when your body cannot digest it properly.

If your body cannot recognise the food, it is like putting diesel into a petrol run car. That explains why I ate less calories by taking off chicken skins and fat, but unfortunately, I still could not lose the weight. When I had no efficient fuel to burn, such as good quality fat, I would feel dizzy and weak whenever I felt hungry. The more frequently I felt hungry, the more times I had to eat during the day. My body continued to take the "burden of digesting the food" without a rest. It is like a carload of weight that burns more fuel, so you have to input more petrol and more often. I was wondering why I had so much weight and fat in my body, including a severe fatty liver condition, which could not convert into fuel to burn when I was hungry?

I believe that many people reading this have had the same questions as I did.

It was because my body functioned at the wrong metabolism, as Charlotte told me. Modern processed foods that I ate and considered healthy, was in fact not at all. I was a highly educated person so I took every advice I could from biology textbooks, main-stream expert/ doctor/ nutritionist opinions, and bought expensive "healthy looking" food and ingredients. I was taught that vegetable oils were healthier to cook with rather than the traditional pork, duck and other animal (saturated) fats that we in the East had been cooking with for millennia. I enjoyed many delicious dishes in the restaurants and never questioned whether these were prepared with good or bad ingredients. This was not in the sphere of my knowledge at that time and I believe that most people are trapped in the same situation as I was.

It was not my fault that I did not want to look after myself: fitness and health. It was not my intention to stay overweight and unhealthy. In fact, I tried very hard most of the time, but got the opposite results. I got every bit of information from my "knowledge pool" wrong, and never did I have a chance to examine it until the day I had that dinner with Paul and Charlotte in London.

Ideally, here I list some guidelines for good food for you to easily follow in your daily meals in Table 4.1:

Table 4.1
Easy to Practice for Ideal Food/ Diet to Lose the Weight
(or back to the right weight)

Key List	Explanation	Check (Y/ N)
More organic food	Your body does not "understand" pesticides, herbicides, chemicals, and they can be very toxic. Organic does not necessarily mean organic "certified", but from your garden, from an ethical farm you are familiar with.	
Stable saturated fat to heat/ cook with	Your body does not "understand" (polyunsaturated) unstable vegetable oil after it is heated into different (or toxic) chemical compounds.	
Less processed food	Your body's metabolism does not always "understand" many artificial ingredients/ flavours in processed food.	
As fresh as possible	Nutrients inside the food decline over time and oxidise.	

	It is not difficult to detect, you can actually taste it.	
Read all the ingredients	Your body does not "understand" many artificial additives/ ingredients in most processed food.	
Fermented food with meals & drink before or after meals	A broad selection of "live" probiotics can provide "fuel" to your gut with a balanced friendly bacteria environment.	
Non-refined natural sugars & real sea salt	Your body "understands" them, and they contain the minerals you need.	
Do not eat all the time	You eat because you "think" you want to eat, or you look at the time you "should" eat? Or you are bored. Use your "gut-feeling", not your head, or by just looking at your watch. Give your body a break! [1]	
Re-examine anything addictive	Why it "makes you crave it" why does it cause you to be addicted to it?	

	e.g., re-fined sugar , refined carbs, deep fried processed foods[2] are designed to cause cravings and addictions. caught up into a vicious cycle.	
Carbohydrates in the last meal/ low-GI better	If you do not want to be hungry often during the day, leave the Carbohydrates in your last meal. Not all carbohydrates make you fat, but if refined they do make you feel hungry easier than fat and protein. *** The Worst: wheat-grain for your breakfast!!! It can make you overweight, easily hungry again, causing you to eat more…then you create a vicious circle which is hard to escape from (like my former self).**	
Avoid alcohols	Thanks to Covid-19… now everyone knows alcohol kills good bacteria, and also, most people realise the importance of gut health is built on a good bacterial environment to digest and absorb food.	

Avoid wheat	Gluten may cause inflammation and keep you bloated. But it also depends whether you are indigenous to the wheat, and how the wheat flour is processed (e.g., sourdough bread is a better choice, as are organic and ancient indigenous grains)	

Source: Dr. I Han

If you are from a rice country like me, I strongly recommend you quit the wheat flour [3]. As I've grown up with most noodle dishes, I did not realise the wheat-based noodles cause the most inflammation in my body which is held as fat in the body. When I completely dropped bread, noodles, dumplings, so many foods made with wheat flour, the weight dropped easily. An old lady I know who owns a very famous rice-cake café in the rural community, is in a very good and solid beautiful shape in her 70s. When I shared my journey, she smiled and said, "of course, I never touch the wheat. I eat rice because it grows here."

I am happy that I don't need to inquire how to lose the weight anymore. I eat happily, with many delicious dishes, and don't feel hungry anymore. I can eat pizza, cakes, bread without wheat (examples in Figure 4.2). I also enjoy deep fried chips (in stable saturated fat) which I could never have in my previous diet. I invited one of my previous MBA students, Sylvani Anggraeni Singhakowinta, to demonstrate how easy it is to make wheat-free brownies with low GI palm sugar in my Food Therapy workshop. She is from Indonesia and has enjoyed inventing many delicious wheat-free recipes for years. The participants in the workshop learned how easy we can make wheat-free brownies, using healthy ingredients (Figure 4.3). More importantly, all participants thought that the brownie was even better tasting than any brownie they had before.

Figure 4.2
Delicious wheat-free bread, pizza, desserts
(natural ingredients only)

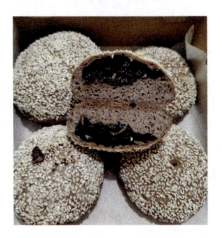

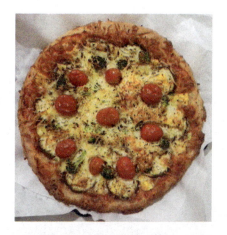

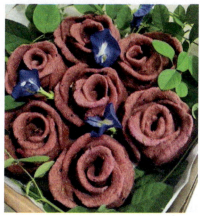

Source: Sylvani Anggraeni Singhakowinta

Figure 4.3
Wheat-free brownie prepared by all the participants in the workshop

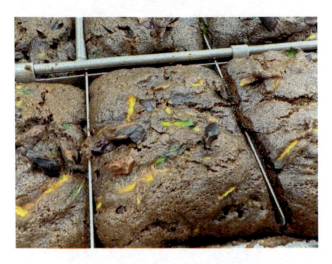

Source: Fen-Hua Liu (one of the workshop participants)

There are two common questions you might ask:
1. Fasting:
   Fasting during the day [see note 2] is not included here. If you did 3+ days, you probably understand how the body fully removes everything in your digestive system in the first 2-3 days. Fasting is not necessary if your only goal is to lose weight. From my point of view, fasting is to give the body a break and to detox the toxins accumulated in our system (e.g., pesticides, chemicals, heavy metals). Fasting can also support weight loss, but it is easy to regain weight back to your normal weight after fasting, or even more, if you return to your old habits by

putting the wrong foods/ ingredients into your mouth.

2. Keto diet:
   The goal of keto diet is to increase metabolism. After my weight was lost to a stable point, I took on a 6-week keto diet in order to burn my body fat more easily. When we had a long history of eating an excess amount of carbohydrates, the body has been trained to burn easy fuel (carbohydrates) and gradually "forgotten" to burn the fat. That was why when I was overweight and carried a lot of fat I was unable to burn. When I was hungry, I was dizzy and shaking, so I had to find sugar or sweets to stop the immediate hunger crisis. I was wondering why I could not burn my body fat while there was an excess there. If your body can easily switch to burn fat rather than burn carbohydrates, the fat will be easily burned when needed. Keto diet can often help people with chronic illnesses, metabolic syndrome and weight loss. As a side note, if you revert to your "usual" bad eating habits, you will regain the weight again easily.

For decades we have been mass educated by trusted authorities and the media that animal fats caused the 3-highs: high blood pressure, high blood fat, high risk of heart attack. However, I always had the issue of high levels of Triglycerides, liver fat, and blood fat when I ate out and used unsaturated vegetable oil to cook with. Many of my friends who are not overweight still had the "3-highs" problem. As soon as I converted to completely avoiding food cooked from vegetable oils, my weight dropped, and my medical reports (including Triglycerides) all went back to normal. Saturated fat (animal fat, coconut oil, Ghee) is a stable fat, which is not easily damaged when exposed to heat. Traditional fats such as ghee and lard and coconut oil are recognised by our body and easily metabolised. One of my friends commented: "No wonder my grandma who always cooked with pork fat never had any 3-highs, but I do, eventhough I use expensive polyunsaturated oil which I thought was good to cook in."

Realistically, it is a choice along the 0-100% spectrum if all ideal food is at the end of the extreme, 100%:

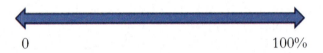

0   100%

If you are a busy person like me, spending 30 minutes to quickly prepare your meal is not a problem, which is roughly about the same amount of time as you wait for a take-away (Figure 4.4). Because you are not hungry all the time, you might just need two or even one good dinner-level dish a day. Sometimes I cook for my large family during the holiday and it usually takes 60 to 90 minutes to prepare dishes for up to 10 people. Just a reminder here dear reader, I rarely cooked before. If now I manage to cook almost every day, I imagine that it should not be a big problem for most of you. If you have more time, you might enjoy spending 2 or 3 hours preparing healthy and delicious dishes.

Figure 4.4
An example of my 30-minute meal:
Scrambled eggs, vegetables, fruits, purple sweet potato pancake

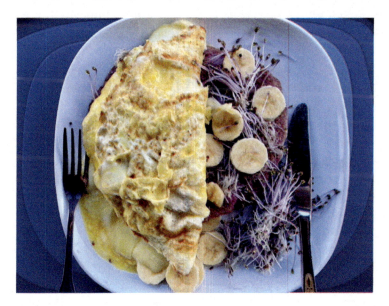

Source: Dr. I Han

Regardless, you do not have to choose 100% correct food/ingredients all the time. However, sometimes it is necessary to eat out with family or friends. There are also other occasions to eat out such as a birthday party. However, it remains a personal choice how closer to 100% you are committed to. For example, when I travel and stay in a hotel, I have no cooking facilities. I then have to find a place to eat, with choices of rice, and I bring my own coconut oil to ask the restaurant to cook with (if the chef was not happy to use my oil or neither does he/ she have a good one, I just simply changed to eat at the other restaurant). When I fly long-haul trip back to Taiwan, I took my own meals [4]. My meals tasted much better than most economy-class meals anyway. It is a personal choice of how much risk exposure you would like to exchange your health/ weight for. Even when eating out, there is always a way to minimise your risk.

Because there have been hundreds of my friends and beyond who are interested in understanding more, I then started a Foundation Course delivered in a 6-week module online on my website (Food Therapy: West Meets East). In addition, there are many invited blogs on the website, including Charlotte Palmer, Paul Sherring, medical doctors, food/ healing practitioners, researchers. An edited book, *Food Therapy: West Meets East*, will be published soon. The purpose is to give more readers the chance to find their own good/ fit way.

The bottom line: do not stick to whatever you learned before, especially if it has never worked for you. Take a view of those delicious food photos by many course participants, posted on my website. You then will get an idea of how many good choices you can have. When you do not feel hungry and still eat a lot of delicious food, including desserts, you will not even think about "cheat days" ever again.

Sustaining blood sugar levels through wise food choices is the best solution to effective weight-loss/ weight-control.

Notes:

[1]
It is not important how many hours are between your meals. There are a lot of books/ courses on intermittent fasting 16-8 (16 hours break window). The purpose is to give your body, or digestive system, a break. Otherwise, when you keep putting the food into your body even when you are not hungry, your digestive system is always overloaded. Thus, even 16-8 is not a good idea. If you eat within 8-hour-window during a day, while the other 16 hours fasting, you might still eat too much during those 8 hours. The simple rule is: no hunger, no eating.

[2]
A known effective way to quit food addiction is dry-fasting [5], or SOD/ enzyme fasting with water. I used to love cakes and sweets too much. After four-day soft dry-fasting (no water, no food, shower/ bath allowed) in 2022, I did not want sweets anymore. In fact, sugar addiction is found as a difficult food addiction to withdraw from [6]. I don't agree, fasting ONLY with water really worked for me, for details refer to [5]. However, I completed a 7-day SOD/ enzyme fasting with water in 2023, in order to repair oxidisation cells (which we all have throughout years).

[3]
Dr William Davis, 2021. *Wheat Belly Total Health*. HarperCollins Publisher: London.

[4]
My typical in-flight meal: stirred-rice with meat and vegetables (1st meal), 6 boiled eggs (4 as the 2nd meal, 2 as snacks), steamed or roasted sweet potatoes (2nd meal).

[5]
Dunning, A. 2020. *The Phoenix Protocol Dry Fasting for Rapid Healing and Radical Life Extension: Functional Immortality.*

[6]
Nicole M. Avena, N.M., Rada P., Hoebel, B.G. 2008. Evidence for sugar addiction: Behavioral and neurochemical effects of intermittent, excessive sugar intake. *Neuroscience & Biobehavioral Reviews*, 32 (1): 20-39.

Commentary

Charlotte Palmer

20+ years as a food specialist
Founder of True Health Talks
London, UK

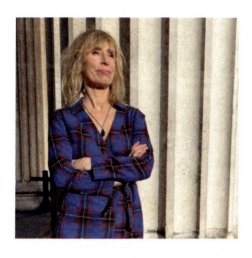

When I first met Dr Han her ideas about food were like many people given by the powerful food industry and not in her own interests. Despite her academic background Dr Han had weight issues that she could not have control over, due to poor dietary choices. Paul and I offered evidence-based lifestyle guidance that went against the grain and the current narrative, but we knew it would help. We watched the transformation of Dr Han over a period of months as she shed the pounds and improved her health and fitness. This book is about her journey to her transformed self.

We all have different metabolic types but most of us are eating foods that either don't suit us or are newly introduced into the human diet. 80% of foods in our supermarkets didn't exist a hundred years ago nor were found in the human diet. Our ancient ancestors had predominantly fat burning metabolisms and we were not hard wired to thrive on refined, modified and processed foods.

For most of human history including much of the 20th Century, insufficient food was the greatest nutritional challenge. To tackle this, governments sought to stimulate the production and distribution of as much inexpensive food as possible, in particular starchy high carbohydrate staple commodities and their shelf stable processed products. At the time a global pandemic of obesity and chronic diseases from the widespread availability of inexpensive unhealthy food was inconceivable. Due to a rise in agriculture the cheap and abundant availability of grains has seeped its way into the modern Western diet wreaking havoc in the populations' health. Processed foods are now commonplace in our diets.

"The nation is literally eating itself into a state of avoidable chronic disease and the government has no policy on prevention." BANT CEO Satu Jackson.

Humans were not designed to metabolise these modern replacements for our ancestral food; the only people they benefit are the food industry. Metabolic syndrome is a rising global health problem due to these global food trends and misinformation is driven purely by profits not for the sake of human health.

Over the past 20 years I have worked with hundreds of cases of metabolic syndrome and helped and supported many to reverse their conditions:

Inflammation, weight issues, thyroid, gut, and heart issues…. for example can all be helped significantly with an ancestrally aligned diet.

Weight loss needs to start with the right mental attitude underpinned with commitment and a good diet plan. The best way to eat healthily is to go back to what your ancestors were eating a few centuries ago. Be as close to that diet as you can. When people ate all of the animal fats and food was in its most natural form.

Seek an expert to guide you through the process and don't believe those 'food industry messages' who prioritise profit over integrity and have no investment in your health.

Many government food authorities and advisory bodies are not fit for purpose and only benefit the food industry this is a great part of the problem and not part of the solution.

Commentary

Jean Chen

Founder of S.J. Sustainability
Health Manager of Health Club
Kaohsiung, Taiwan

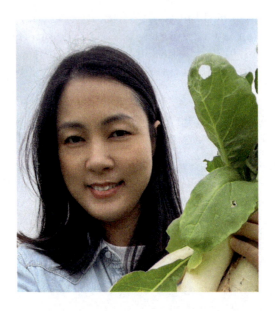

I am one of Dr. Han's witnesses from her overweight time to her weight loss transformation. As I asked her, I was amazed that she did not control her diet by counting calories. Of course she did not take any tablets, surgery, or medical solutions to lose her weight significantly. She eats the right food/ ingredients, with only limited exercise (not including the weight training in the latter stage).

I was one of Dr. Han's friends who wanted to know how she managed to lose over 15 kilograms in about a year, and became healthier!

I signed up for her online 6-week with other participants. She put her lessons into a course because she was "lazy" to tell one friend at a time. Thanks to her educational profession, we had a chance to examine our food and diet, and try for ourselves.

I was very interested in a real experiment and chance to become healthier. I did not have a problem with my weight, but I had issues with bloating and gastroesophageal reflux for decades. I'd tried many medical solutions (amongst which Western and Chinese) for many years. None of them worked.

By the second week of the course, I noticed that my gut bloating problem improved significantly! Also, other symptoms such as gastroesophageal reflux disappeared.

The major change in me during these six weeks was to quit my favourite wheat-noodle dish with traditional Taiwanese sesame sauce, which I used to eat almost every other day. I mostly avoided food with wheat during this course. I then realised that wheat was something my body didn't need or benefit from!

Therefore, I tried other wheat-free ingredients to make delicious "noodle" dishes for me and my family. I also made many other East/ West dishes, such as radish cakes, meat dumplings, and meatballs for the scallion pancakes, pan-fried dumplings, and boiled dumplings, without any ingredients that are not allowed.

The other important lesson is to use ONLY a good source of fats and proteins. I used to buy high-priced vegetable oils which I (and many other people) thought were good. But I was wrong. Only saturated fat is safe to cook with, it will not convert to toxic chemical compounds for our cells, that simply are unable to recognize them.

That was suddenly an Ah-ha moment for me. I did not understand that many elderly people from my grandparent's generation cooked with pork fat but stayed healthy until old age . On the contrary, we live in the "advanced" modern world where we start to become ill as early as our thirties.

Now, I make most of my breakfast and dinner at home (Figure 4.5). I cut down eat-out occasions in order to avoid toxic vegetable oils and unnecessary ingredients. There are so many hidden ingredients actually harming us that we take for granted.

Figure 4.5
Typical breakfast I cook for my family:
wheat-free sandwiches/ bagels, scrambled eggs, yogurt, fruit & tea

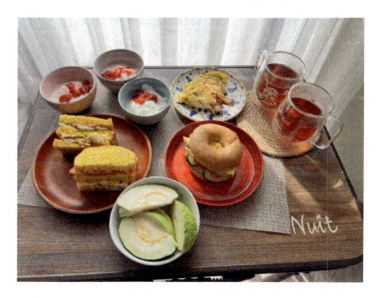

Source: Jean Chen

Simple rule: we eat only those food/ ingredients that positively support (or the bottom line: don't harm) our bodies. I will definitely continue this journey as my lifestyle. Those friends and family around me also witnessed my transformation and started to follow me. Once it becomes a habit, metabolism will naturally level out. Finally, I would like to thank Dr. Han for selflessly sharing her own journey by putting all this precious information now into this book.

Chapter 5

Chinese Medical Training: A Holistic View

This chapter aims at establishing a holistic view towards our body. Weight loss and muscle strength certainly play a part in physical holistic health. In turn, a journey towards holistic health is an integrative process to establish and support your ideal weight and muscle strength (Figure 8.1).

People in Taiwan like to ask whether Chinese medicine is better than Western medicine, or vice versa.

Western medicine (allopathic) is a singular-formula treating one symptomatic problem at a time, while Chinese medicine is a compound treating multiple symptoms at a time via the root cause. This is a very simple answer neither is better or worse, quoting my friend with a doctoral degree working as a R&D head of a world-famous pharmaceutical company based in Boston. In terms of long term health issues Naturopathic medicine addresses the root cause, allopathic medicine only suppresses and alleviates symptoms.

Growing up with Western medical treatments, I used to view Chinese medicine as unscientific. I did not trust Chinese doctors, as many of them looked archaic, not located in modern buildings, and most of them seemed mysterious to me. When my mother took me to a Chinese doctor to heal my wounded legs from exercise, I joked about the medical patches referring to them as "dog-skin medical patch (狗皮膏藥), or herbal compress" as they were dark in colour with a special smell. It wasn't until my forties when I learned more about the constraints of my father's medical conditions, while he was treated in one of the top western hospitals in Taipei. did I then realise his multiple dysfunctions would eventually be the cause of his death even long before he passed away.

"How could anyone accuse Chinese medicine of a lack of scientific basis, given thousands of years of human experiences? How many years do we carry our human body tests now?" I was reminded by my Boston friend who worked in a big pharmaceutical company. "Anything you cannot prove does not mean it is not scientific, nor does it not exist."

Western doctors treat one dysfunction at a time, just as their training and medicines were designed for. It was not their problem. As I discussed my father's case with my Boston friend, he also agreed that western doctors would have limitations when dealing with multiple dysfunctions.

Alternatively, Chinese medical philosophy views the human body from a holistic view. A lower back pain can be caused by the mis-alignment in the other part of the body [1]. A kidney dysfunction can also cause hormonal imbalance and sexual dysfunction.

I am not a medical doctor, but I have participated in various experimental competitions, including physics, chemistry, and biology, from elementary school to high school. I understand the basic rules in the laboratory. In Taiwan, I was waived the entrance examinations twice. I entered Taipei First Girls' Senior High School and later the Department of Physics at National Taiwan University because of my outstanding achievements in conducting laboratory research in Physics while still in high school.

The science in the laboratory is to test ONE variable at a time while controlling all else equally.

For example, I've conducted many experiments in teas because of my social enterprise business. Figure 5.1 is one of the examples of how to do a pH test on teas. When the pH is the variable that we would like to test in teas (red), other variables (blue) have to be controlled, including the temperature to brew the tea, tea brewing time, types of tea (loose leaves, same variety of tea trees), so we can observe the pH results among oolong tea leaves, red tea leaves, and green tea leaves. Thus, we can conclude whether oolong tea has a higher pH than red and green teas. In other words, we cannot use different types of tea trees between oolong, red, and green tea. Neither can we brew the teas at different temperatures or time, even when I normally recommend customers to brew green tea at a lower temperature, while oolong tea needs more brewing time.

This test cannot be used to generalised other types of tea tree varieties to prove oolong tea has a higher pH than red or green tea. Neither can it be generalised to cold-brew teas. In the same way, a laboratory experiment is completely different from our daily lives. The map is not the territory.

Figure 5.1
Laboratory Test:
The Case of pH Test on Teas

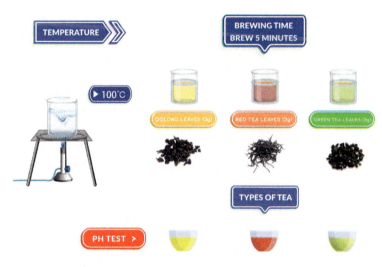

Source: Livy Sung

The earlier years of solid training in scientific laboratory experiments, plus my doctoral methodology training in social science, all aided in my current understanding of research journal papers in nutrition, food, traditional medicine/ therapy, and Western biochemistry and pharmaceuticals.

How is this "science" even close to our humanity? There must be a broad scope of assumptions and controls in order to observe the variable the researcher wishes to study. All academic studies tell readers the assumptions, methodology, findings, and the limitations (boundary conditions). We cannot just grab the conclusion of a research paper and apply it to the real world. That is so wrong!!!

In current times, most of our information is fed to us by trusted authorities, governments and industry professionals. In the majority of cases mis-information is delivered due to vested interests and hidden financial incentives.

Relevant so-called "professional advice" that we get daily from friends, social media, or newspapers, such as "there is a doctor who once said that poor diet is the root cause of most cancers." Whilst we might gather useful bits of knowledge from various sources, we often still don't get the big picture, or a practical understanding of how the whole body system works and how to apply that to a specific issue we want to improve.

Our modern culture has taught us to formulate an opinion without examining the evidence. We rely upon the media and the government to spoon feed us information. This is a global problem due to the focus on economics instead of human health, and information is not evidence based because it does not benefit the food and agriculture industry. One of the many examples:

"One common modern belief by many mainstream health professionals is that saturated (animal fats) causes high cholesterol which in turn lead to a heart attack." this standpoint has never been proven and is based on shaky foundations due to a widespread support for the theory by Dr Ancel Keys in the 1950s that saturated fat causes cardiovascular disease (CVD). This was based on his famous 24 country theoretical study, which he cherry picked to fit his theory. "At the same time a nutritionist said that it was sugar not fat, that caused obesity, but he was ignored. This was the beginning of a long held global food myth."

For decades we have been asking what the real cause of weight gain is?

As many public agencies tell us, it is an excess of calories and too much dietary fat. So why are we dealing with a global health crisis as metabolic syndrome is on an alarming rise?

There was another recent social media spread:
"Recent research found that vitamin C & K will actually cause cancer cells to grow…"
……..
Is this really true or just speculation?

I always go back to check the origin:
1. Who exactly made that statement?
2. Is there any original research papers published in the related topics to support point 1?
3. If yes, find the paper and read what was written in the papers? What was the methodology? What were the variables they controlled? What were the constraints (research limitations)?

Only if points 1 and 3 can be verified, we will be able to understand how the experimental findings might be applied and under what conditions onto the real-world cases. This is how we have been trained in all (social or natural) scientific doctoral programmes in research design, research method, and research implications/limitations. This rigorous training in conducting research and its application is particularly useful when examining in the social complex world, as small as individual human beings, and as large as collective social groups at many different levels in practice. That's why a PhD like me is always cautious whenever I receive any information before I distribute it or apply it.

The human body is a complex biological system. From a holistic view, an individual human being is not only living on its own, but also living with other human beings, species, plants,.... in a surrounded holistic environment [2]. It is a "small universe" within a "big universe" as told in many ancient Chinese medicine books. I would like to borrow the complexity theory when I invited one of the book editors of *Handbook of Research Methods in Complexity Science*, Mr. Christopher Day, to provide a speech for my MBA students. Mr. Day talked about the complexity situation among countries. He also asked every student to participate in a game outside the classroom, with complexity movement. The complexity of the world at different levels simply describes the concept of holistic view of Chinese medical training here: a slight move will affect everything else, or "pull one hair and the whole body moves" as the Chinese saying goes.

The human body is very complicated, but it is in fact very simple:
Balance!

In other words:
Any unbalanced condition causes the problem. [3]

Unlike the principles of single-variable experiments in Western medicine, the holistic view examines the human, as a small universe, *i.e.*, an entirety, which is a part of a large universe around us.

Thus, there are a lot of confusions without a holistic view. For examples:
"I have a ginger shot every morning. I think that is good for me."
Correct: Ginger is good, which has been used as "medicinal introductory (藥引), or facilitator" in many Chinese medicine compound.
Danger: But ginger on its own is a heating food, which will balance if you have a cold body, but not a hot/ warm one.

"My (Western) doctor told me that green tea is good for my father's cancer."
Correct: Green tea is good for its antioxidants in general. For an existing cancer case, general green tea is probably not enough to help, except in high concentration form [4].
Danger: However, if drinking normal green tea, which is "a cold attribute" in food, many cancer patients might already become weak in condition. Therefore, maybe red tea from the Chinese medical point of view will help to boost Qi and warm up the weak body, while red tea still contains a good level of antioxidants [5].

Many natural ingredients might contain many good attributes to human health, but without considering individual body condition. Consider taking something known as good, that same good thing, despite its reputation and all that is deemed good may not be compatible with your specific body, or could have an unexpected interaction (good, bad, or neutral). The best strategy, however, is by controlling variables as you can, like the principle in a laboratory, and only observing effects from ONE single variable at a time. By doing so, you will be able to research yourself and understand your own body to cope with a holistic solution over time.

I received an Auricular certification from World Federation of Chinese Naturopathy (Figure 5.2). Our ears are a miniature of our whole-body condition. It is a truly holistic application on diagnosis and treatment. I started to realise this holistic view of the human body as a small universe, and that there is another smaller universe of our ears. They tell whether you are healthy, whether any part of your body has been suffering some problem, or even foresee it.

Figure. 5.2
Certified Auricular course
Dr. Li & Chairman Dr. Shih of
World Federation of Chinese Naturopathy

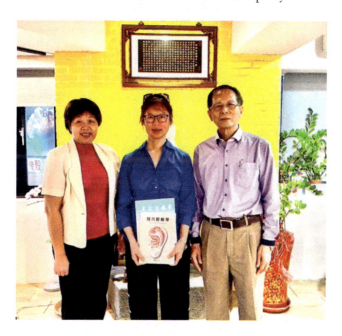

Source: Dr. I Han

It's not a laughing matter that it's better not to show your pictures with ears on social media if you do not like other people knowing your health condition. When watching a film, it was very interesting to read many male ears which I shared with my family about their health conditions I observed.

After I obtained the certification, I did many practices among my university colleagues, my friends and family. It was an initial step towards understanding how Chinese doctors do their jobs:

"See, smell/ hear, ask, cut (-through) (望聞問切)"

i.e., see their ears, diagnose by asking whether they don't feel alright in a specific spot and observe that there might be something not right, and they feedback to you (either confirm it or reject it). This is an iterative process to build on your own practice over time. When I achieved 50 practised cases, I was more experienced than just sitting in the lectures. I also built even more experience from the cases by joining Dr. Wen-yu Li's volunteering road trip, where I could see hundreds of ears during a day. It's a learning process with a good mentor to advise and make progress overtime.

The most impressive experience was when I looked at one of my family member's ears and asked if she had a problem. She denied it, but came back to me two days later to confirm that she found out I was right. Later, Dr. Li taught me that ears also tell whether it is a recent problem (including my family's case, i.e., she did not feel it until later, but it already happened) or has been an old problem for quite a long time.

Two years later, I had a chance to learn the pulse measure/ diagnosis with a very senior Chinese doctor, Dr. Mingchen Lin, in Taichung. Dr. Lin's pulse theory and practice goes beyond the human body. The pulse is the show of energy, which is inside a human body, outside a human body, even outside our planet. All these sources of energy together influence one another, regardless of their distance, strong or weak, natural or artificial. The energy influences the function of organs, circulations (Qi and blood) at the physical level and beyond (mental and spiritual levels).

There was a patient who came in and said that she could not sleep for days, always hearing sounds of waves during the night. After Dr. Lin's diagnosis, he told the lady, it was normal to hear those sounds. When he went to Tibet on a medical volunteer trip, a lot of monks, or She-Fu (師傅, masters in the temple) had very similar experiences from time to time. The patient was then relaxed. It is also another placebo effect as well:)

Pulse is another holistic teller of the whole-body condition. Cut (切) means to touch the body and get more information, where the pulse tells very comprehensive information. Dr. Lin's five-section pulse method (五段脈) provides a patient's condition in details with four levels of pressure on the wrist. The first-depth might show a cold body attribute while the fourth-depth might turn to a heat attribute. The human body is simple as well as complicated. It is simple because if there is something stuck or not in balance, it causes a problem sooner or later. It is complicated because an ill patient can be hot and cold at the same time, and it can vary from organs to organs. However, it is not that difficult to understand:

If an area is blocked, there must be some area colder while other places are on fire. Therefore, there is no one single formula as in Western medicine to cure everyone even with the same symptom because everyone is different in terms of their body condition.

It is a very important initial holistic view to understand the patient in each case. During several real practice situations in Dr. Lin's Chinese Clinics, I studied more directly with Dr.

Lin in how to diagnose and treat a patient by using Chinese herbal medicine. In his clinics, however, cupping (Ba Guan, 拔罐) and acupuncture are also available, but I have not yet had a chance to learn them.

You did not actually need a "certification" in the past, if you have a good mentorship from the old-fashioned traditional approach used for thousands of years. "Being ill for long makes you become a good doctor (久病成良醫)", as an old Chinese saying told, because of the accumulated experiences possessed by each individual case, *i.e.*, you know yourself the best. Traditionally, there had always been a system of mentorship and medical family successions in the Chinese world throughout generations and thousands of years, which produced competent healers.

Notes:
[1]
Other than Chinese medicine, later on I found Western osteopathy, and many traditional medicines/ therapies took the similar holistic view.

[2]
Upcoming book: **_Quantum Energy: Physics and Beyond_**

[3]
Refer to many ancient Chinese classics readings: *I Ching, Yellow Emperor's Classic of Internal Medicine, Cold Damage* (Zhang Zhongjing's *Shanghan Zabing Lun*),......

[4]
Refer to Food Therapy West Meets East/ blog article: High Concentration Green Tea for Blood Circulation

[5]
Some tea plants, such as Red Jade (Taiwan No.18), contains even higher levels of antioxidant than most green tea, despite being processed into fully fermented red tea, according to a laboratory experiment, as shown in Figure 5.3.

Figure 5.3 Experiment Result: Antioxidant in Teas

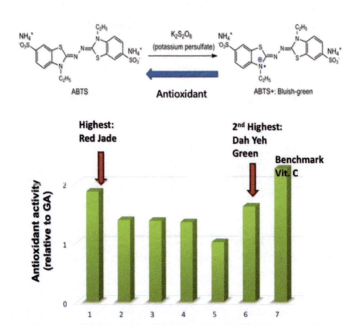

Source: Formosan Farms (Figure 1 in the blog: *Antioxidants in Teas*)

Commentary

Dr Wen-Yu Li

Managing Director of Lai-Yu-An Chinese Medical Clinics
President of Taichung Academy of Chinese Doctor
Association
Taichung, Taiwan

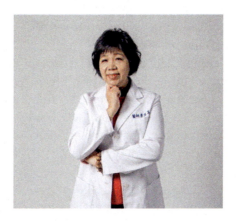

Dr. Han is a humble and smart student. I met her at my speech of "Big World of Small Ears", an introduction to Auricular diagnosis for members of the World Federation of Chinese Naturopathy. After that, she was very interested in studying more Auricular diagnosis and treatment. She participated in the certified course held by the World Federation of Chinese Naturopathy three-day intensive course and received her certification. After that, she worked very hard to practise with friends and colleagues, also discussed with me from time to time. I found that she had a good understanding and analysis of what those cases were about. She also shared what those friends and colleagues gave as positive feedback after her practiced treatment. I then invited her to join my volunteer clinic tours in Taiwan. In the first two tours, she watched how I diagnosed and treated patients within a day. In the later tours, she started to practise Auricular diagnosis and treatment under my supervision.

According to the Chinese medicine concept of meridians, Auricular diagnosis and treatment is using the messages in ears as a whole reflection of the body (生物全息律). There are many acupuncture-points in a small ear. Those points represent an up-side-down body, just like an unborn baby, with head down and hip up. We don't have to use invasive needles for Auricular acupuncture. In the course, I teach students to use Dr. Li-Chun Huang's books and practice with non-invasive stickers, each sticker with a small magnetic ball on the acupuncture point to stimulate and treat (Figure 5.4).

Auricular treatment can be easily applied and work effectively. The non-invasive magnetic ball can be carried outside the clinic, which means longer practice (I usually advise my patients to take it off in 3 to 7 days after treatment) than a needle. In my Chinese clinic, it works really well in improving insomnia, excessive dreaming, motion sickness, tinnitus, digestion, trachea, obesity, and releasing various pains. It is easy to treat, long lasting (take-home), with almost no side effects.

There were many amazing cases in our volunteer medical tours. First was an Indian born patient with CP (Cerebral palsy). When I put Auricular stickers on his ears, he immediately could relax his both hands which he could never do before. Second was a Malaysian who could not open his left eye because of Nasopharyngeal cancer. When I put Auricular stickers on his ears, he immediately could open his left eye. The other case was a Taiwanese passenger on the plane from Taipei to New York who was afflicted by a stroke, or brain stem haemorrhage. I used Auricular treatment and he was able to fly back to Taiwan without requiring other medical treatment upon landing in New York.

Auricular diagnosis/ treatment has been recognised as the easiest entry to learn Chinese medicine/ healing. It is not always necessary to use needles to improve the illness.

Figure 5.4
Auricular Diagnosis & Treatment:

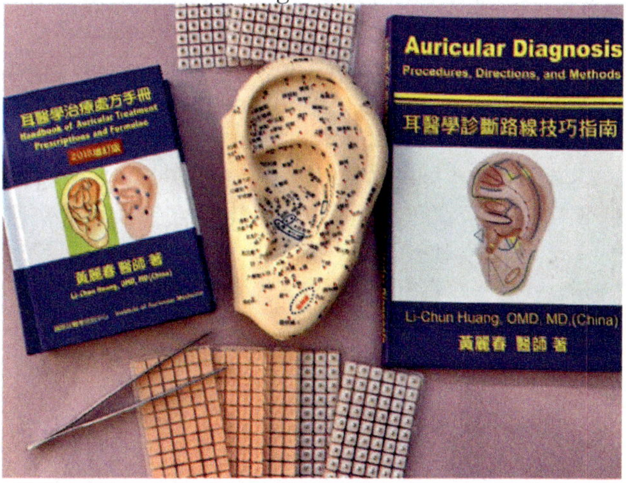

Source: Dr. I Han

Chapter 6

Pai Da Gong: The Easiest Exercise

I used to think of Qi Gong as an elderly-person's exercise. I was so wrong!

The slow movement does not mean it is an easier exercise than other fast-moving ones. Slow movement of Qi Gong exercise, in fact, requires more muscle strength to hold the posture for a longer time. It helps to create a high level of resistance over time.

I started my Qi Gong journey by doing the Qi-Gong-8-Brocades. I did it every morning and started to feel Qi flow after a whole year of daily practice (Figure 6.1). In the beginning, it was not easy to hold those postures with slow movement. That was the first time when I changed my misguided view of Qi Gong for old people only. However, the slow movement of Qi Gong might be less likely to cause damage to elderly people compared with other fast-moving exercises, if they are not fit to practise them (refer to Chapter 7).

Figure. 6.1
Qi-Gong-8-Brocades every morning

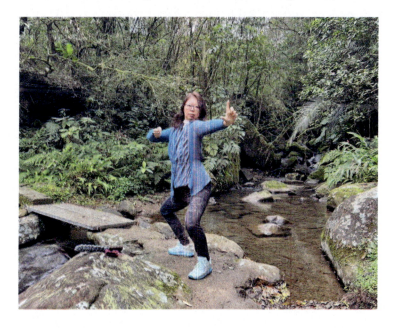

Source: Dr. I Han

Qi has been recognised as flowing energy, equally important as blood circulation to keep the human body functioning and alive. In the recent Western medical point of view, Dr. Yang Jwing-ming highlighted that Qi was possibly more akin to bioelectricity, life-force energy, inside the human body [1]. Tyler (2017) reviewed research in wounded healing of bioelectricity generative processes [2]. Doing Qi Gong every morning does help my body (not just my head) to wake up at the beginning of a day.

When I moved to England in 2019, the weather was too cold for me, compared to the tropical zone of Taiwan. I started to practise Pai Da Gong as an add-on exercise. Pai Da Gong is another easy conditioning of Qi Gong, to boost Qi circulation and help my body warm-up, not just wake-up.

I learned Pai Da Gong from a master, Carol Lai, in Taiwan. She used Pai Da Gong to heal many health issues, including insomnia, digestive problems, menstrual pain, headaches, depression, and muscle pains. The tapping by using a good tool (usually a stick, or bamboo) throughout meridian pathways [3] in a certain sequence and rhythm, creates immediate energy by pushing Qi circulation and unblocking any blockage (Figure 6.2).

Figure.6.2
Pai Da Gong is easy to learn & practice

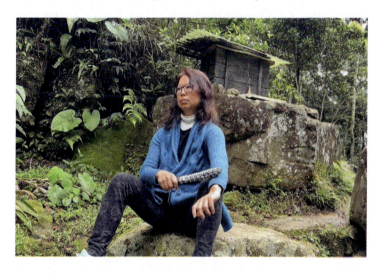

Source: Dr. I Han

The simple philosophy behind this thousand-year-old easy-Qi-Gong is no pain if there is no blockage, and no blockage no illness (通則不痛、通則不病). On the other hand, if there is pain, there is a blockage. Then Pai Da Gong helps to remove/ release it.

Many of my friends and family in Taiwan also took my recommendations to start practising Pai Da Gong because of its ease and instant benefits. For example, my mum practices Pai Da Gong almost every day over the past two years. She had a mobility problem since her childhood. That problem made it very difficult to do any exercise regularly. Pai Da Gong allowed her to not only stand but even sit easily. Two years ago, she was scheduled to have surgery on her knees, but eventually she did not need to go to the surgery after she greatly improved by doing Pai Da Gong, especially when I taught her to spend more time on the area around her knees. I told her to focus on the places where she feels the most pain. It is truly a dilemma:

The more painful the area, the minimum you wish to touch it.
In Pai Da Gong theory, it is, however, the opposite!

You have to tap the place you feel the pain and work through the pain. As long as you can take the pain, it will not hurt you. So, if you are not a qualified healer, never use Pai Da Gong on any other people.

After the Covid-19 lockdown in England, I applied for funds from Active Essex Programme (2021 and 2022) to offer this easy exercise free courses in our local ageing centre (Figure 6.3). Pai Da Gong is so easy to learn and practice, but most people have never heard of it. There was a Qi Gong/ Tai Chi course in the centre. That teacher told me that he never thought Pai Da Gong could be taught. My personal assessment is that once you learn this you can practise at home anytime anywhere. Why strain or spend money to go to a Pai Da Gong class?!

Figure 6.3
Pai Da Gong class in the local ageing centre
Essex, England

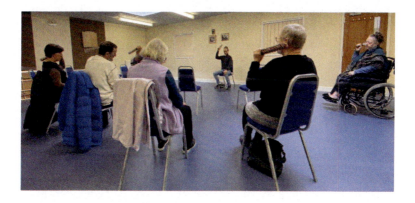

Source: Dr. I Han

Eventually, the immediate energy and health benefits the participants experienced became the motivation to introduce more friends and family to join. During the courses, we as well as the participants experienced the progress, including the colour of their faces (better circulation), the re-activation of muscle energy or even disabled conditions (Figure 6.4). We acknowledge Active Essex Fund to provide the seed of an opportunity in Essex. Because of so much positive feedback from Pai Da Gong participants in the centre [4], I then launched an official Pai Da Gong website in order to help more people in need. It does not matters how old you are or how fit you are. Pai Da Gong always helps Qi/ energy circulation through a rhythm vibrating tapping movement. It boosts the energy by stimulating circulation throughout the body. Pai Da Gong builds another milestone as a healthy lifestyle. I am very excited to share the most effective way to other people in need, especially for many unhealthy people, including my mum, who has always seen physical activity as hard to practise regularly.

For healthy and active people, I found that Pai Da Gong helps to create muscle resistance. When I finally got a chance to go to the gym (see Chapter 7), it certainly helped me to recover faster from weight training and make effective progress.

Figure 6.4
Hand-written thank note from a participant

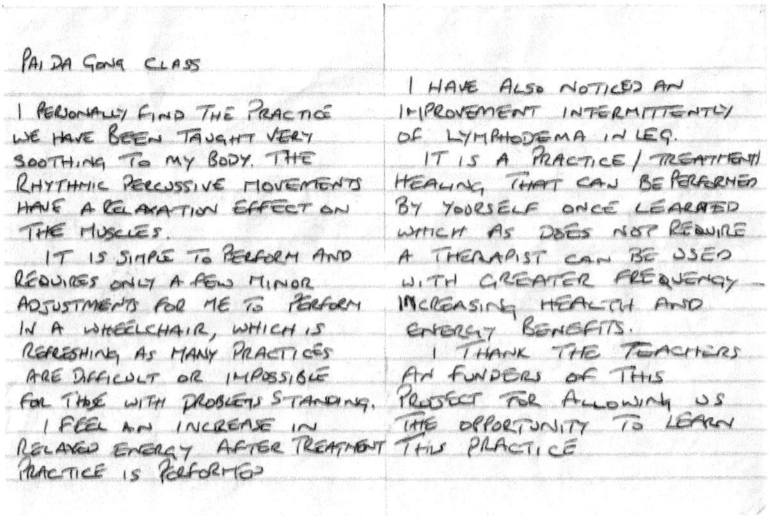

> PAI DA GONG CLASS
>
> I personally find the practice we have been taught very soothing to my body. The rhythmic percussive movements have a relaxation effect on the muscles.
>
> It is simple to perform and requires only a few minor adjustments for me to perform in a wheelchair, which is refreshing as many practices are difficult or impossible for those with problems standing.
>
> I feel an increase in relaxed energy after treatment practice is performed.
>
> I have also noticed an improvement intermittently of lymphodema in leg.
>
> It is a practice/treatment healing, that can be performed by yourself once learned which as does not require a therapist can be used with greater frequency increasing health and energy benefits.
>
> I thank the teachers an funders of this project for allowing us the opportunity to learn this practice.

Source: one of 2021 Active Essex Pai Da Gong course participants

Notes:
[1]
Yang, Jwing-ming. 1992. *Chinese qigong massage: General massage*. Quality Books Inc.: Hong Kong

[2]
Tyler, Sheena E.B. 2017. Nature's electric potential: A systematic review of the role of bioelectricity in wound healing and regenerative processes in animals, humans, and plants. *Frontiers in Physiology*, Vol. 8, Article 627.

[3]
Only in some places such as the neck and kidneys it cannot be applied. Also, I personally don't recommend the tapping method on the head. Instead, I use the stick to massage rather than tap in many places.

[4]
Examples of testimonials (quote from clients and students):

"Noticeable improvement with 1st class."

"Noticed a big difference in my health."

"Excellent practice."

"I can't wait to join the class every week."

"It regenerates me."
"It is absolutely easy to do this exercise."

"I can walk more without sitting down and much faster."

"I feel a flow of energy."

"It is really good to keep me active during the rest of the day (after the course)."

"It certainly helps my circulation, especially my feet."

"I can sit or lay in bed to do this exercise."

Commentary

Carol Lai

10+ years as a Pai Da Gong Healer
Taichung, Taiwan

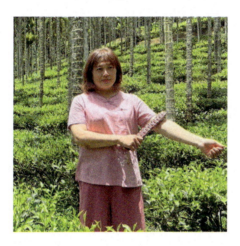

"As a meridian aromatherapist, I have been applying the Pai Da Gong method to my healing process for more than 10 years. I met Dr. Han during one of my Pai Da Gong lessons. She was one of the students. She was volunteering as my patient model for the demonstration purpose in the class with more than 50 other students. She definitely possesses a passion for learning and doing. That's why, I guess, she could apply it very well later in her own interpretation during her ongoing practice, in combination with her teaching profession as a University Professor.

Dr. Han experienced instant effects from my Pai Da healing demonstration. Therefore, she took this method to England and practised it on a day-to-day basis. She asked me questions from time to time about what she learned from Pai Da Gong benefits throughout the time. She then launched an easy-to-learn and easy-to-do module in order to teach other people to do Pai Da Gong exercise themselves at home during the Covid-19 Pandemic lockdown. I was extremely amazed by one of her Pai Da Gong courses in Taiwan in 2022. She extended the method to muscle resistance and strength building, on top of meridian pathways as the common traditional application.

Pai Da Gong will normally cause pain, as no pain no gain. If you practise as a daily exercise, it is safe if the pain is within your tolerance. Pai Da Gong, within your own personal tolerance, can help to activate the muscles and bones, promote body metabolism, and restore the body to a good state.

Pai Da Gong is simple, but the key is to build it into your daily routine to maintain health. If you experience a problem in a specific spot, I recommend you to stay on it and its surrounding area for more time, between 5 to 20 minutes. The principle is to promote the movement of muscle knots, unblock stuck Qi in meridian pathways, by using the tapping method with vibration. According to traditional Chinese medicine (TCM), almost all illnesses are caused by the blockage of Qi. When Pai Da Gong relieves the pain of the blockage, it eventually leads back to good health.

The most common case I treated is long-term pain caused by external force injuries, such as falls, car accidents, and work strains. Pai Da Gong can be used to relieve injury pain. I had a case of a young lady who was suffering from a major injury in a car accident. Her footsteps were small with a challenge to move freely. She was unable to squat or stand to put on her pants. She used four-leg crutches to walk. She lived far away, so only came for treatment once a month. After three times Pai Da Gong treatment, she only needed to use a pair of crutches to support her (Figure 6.5). Also, she recovered her muscles in her buttocks. My Pai Da Gong treatment on her started from the bladder meridian by massaging first, then stretching the tendons, and finally tap straight. In the beginning it was really painful, but through perseverance she improved and the pain was relieved.

Figure 6.5
The car accident case: Improvement of legs pictures on the 1st (right), 2nd (middle), and 3rd time (left) of my treatment

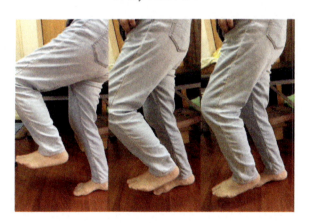

Source: Carol Lai

In addition to physical treatment, Pai Da Gong is also a great method to regulate the mind. It calms down the mind and the body will naturally feel better. After Pai Da Gong treatment or exercise, it is important to smoothen the Qi. It offers a kind of comfort and releases the end of the turbid Qi channel, so that the body will not feel stuck or feel swollen, painful or blocked in certain places.

Pai Da Gong is indeed, a course with a simple concept, and an idea changes a life!

Commentary

Dominique Mannel

Founder of Pai Da Gong African Chapter
Cape Town, South Africa

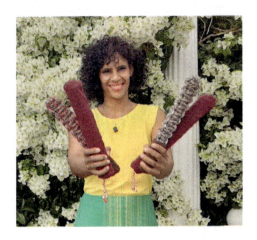

I am a busy mum, a working woman, while dedicating my time towards health-&-fitness, my family and friends, my spirituality, my mental state and quality of life.

As a traveller I used to live in many countries, and I am still exploring new places and spaces. Before returning to South Africa, I lived in Germany for three years. I noticed that by living in Germany with its long winters, I needed to find ways to generate heat, keep strong, fit and healthy. That is when a mutual friend introduced me to Dr. Han. I wanted to be part of the Pai Da Gong Education because it was a decision driven by my passion for holistic learning, holistic living, and personal growth.

My training experience and subsequent classes under the guidance of Dr. Han were incredibly enriching. It focused on practical applications and hands-on experience while giving me insight to Chinese medicine, Qi Gong and our bodies. The support and mentorship provided by Dr. Han was instrumental in shaping my teaching approach. I then became the first certified Pai Da Gong instructor in the EU.

Pai Da Gong, a profound source of ancient wisdom, has found its way to the vibrant landscapes of South Africa, when I opened a studio in Paarl in June 2023. This blend of ancient teachings and contemporary methods creates a distinctive niche, catering to individuals seeking a well-rounded approach to physical, mental, and spiritual well-being. Although Pai Da Gong is good for all age-groups, I find that my elderly clients benefit from it the most. Their common feedback:

It is easy to do, they do not require any additional space to do it, and they feel energised immediately.

To the readers considering Pai Da Gong, I encourage you to embrace this opportunity wholeheartedly. In closing, I extend my gratitude to Dr. Han for her unwavering support and wisdom. To the readers, I wish you a transformative and enlightening experience with Pai Da Gong – where every lesson learned becomes a stepping stone toward a brighter, healthier and thus more fulfilling future.

Chapter 7

Weight Training: The Muscle Strength

My greatest barrier to the gym was that I didn't like the sight of big muscle men or women. I did not enjoy watching fitness/ muscle/ bodybuilder competitions (*i.e.*, 健美先生小姐) on the TV. I never expected myself to be even remotely close to any of them, not in this lifetime.

Going to the gym occurred as hard work; observing many people in the gym (there have been built-in gyms in business/ residential buildings since the early 2000s in Taiwan), they looked exhausted and not a pleasant sight. Going to a gym seemed like a "big" thing to most people I saw and knew. They wanted to "exercise" but they had to take on a strenuous workout in the gym which put me off.

I was wondering how they can make it happen on a regular basis?!

My initial thought was: probably NOT!

Many of my friends made the decision to start an exercise regime at the gym, and purchased 20 or 30 course vouchers with a large chunk of their own money. By investing their cash, they hoped it might "help" them to achieve their fitness goals. But, later on, I found that very few of them fully expended all the vouchers.

"It's too hard to continue"
"I am too lazy to show up on a regular basis"
"I'm too tired to go after my job"
And so on, many similar excuses I had heard throughout the years.

My friend used to tease me: "Doing old people Qi-Gong exercise is not good. You should be like me: run marathons." [1]

Firstly, it was common to say Qi-Gong is an elderly person's exercise, as I had such a misguided judgement when I was young. The reason I guess, though, was probably because it is a "slow" movement, which most elders can handle well, while it is not easy for them to do "fast" movement exercise as a routine (refer to Chapter 6). But, even Qi-gong is a slow movement, I then realised it is hard core when I started to practise Qi-Gong-8-Brocades and Pai Da Gong. The many old Chinese Gong practices train in resistance of the body, which requires stable muscle/ bone to hold the position far longer than running.

Secondly, I did not like to run because my legs are thin (and weak, if without training), which made me feel pain. I did not want to take the risk of damaging my legs, knees, and feet.

However, my misconceptions about exercise were completely "destroyed" when I met Mr. Universe/ World Championship holder Ian Dowe at Dowe Dynamics Gym in London. His legacy since the 1970s has seen him develop and train many champions by his so-called "old school" method in the modern world. Eight weeks of training with Ian, between April and June 2023, entirely changed my view of the gym!

Ian Dowe has developed a very simple but effective formula: exercise, rest, and eat [2].

Nothing else.

It was not hard at all, even for me as a green beginner.

Once committed, to my surprise I made significant progress even in the first two weeks. My osteopath Benjamin Pluke checked my body condition in the second week. He was amazed at how my muscles had developed and came back to life, which had never been the case in the past three years on this journey. By the seventh week of my training with Ian, Benjamin confirmed that my overall body condition became younger.

These 8-week training was absolutely not the "week of hell" (地獄週) I was expecting (as in the Marine Corps or similar boot camps), or was warned against by many of my male friends in England and in Taiwan. Instead, three days a week did not discourage me from attending, and it even became a pleasant routine. I did not feel at all challenged, did not feel tired or any muscle pain after the workout, instead I gained the benefits of :

- ✓ Increased fitness level…the first four weeks
- ✓ Increased muscle strength…the following four weeks

It was not a miracle!

This is how your gym workout should be, as Mr. Universe Ian Dowe taught me.

Ian Dowe has been a British legacy for over four decades. His accolades include :
- Mr. Universe, NABBA (1977, 81, 82)
- World Amateur Championships, IFBB (1983, 84, 86, 87, 2001, 2003, 2004, 2005)
- European Championships, WABBA (1977, 80, 82), IFBB (1984, 96, 2003)
- Mr Britain, NABBA (1970, 78,79, 80, 81, 82)

He worked and shared the same methodology with Arnold Schwarzenegger and Joe Weider in the 1960-70s.

What's the secret?

Workout aligned within your own Comfort Zone*.

Let me revisit the definition of 'comfort zone', which was explained at the beginning of this book:

It does not mean anything negatively: within your own limits and comfort, no stress.
It is a dynamic concept.
In the short term, your 'comfort zone' moves up and down according to your own physical and mental condition.
In the long term, your 'comfort zone' evolves and eventually shifts to the next level.

The 'Comfort Zone' rule makes the fastest improvement in fitness, in muscle strength, and in recovery.
Two major benefits:

1. The 'Comfort Zone' keeps you away from potential damage, which is definitely the goal for anyone who is looking to get healthier and stronger by attending a gym.
2. The 'Comfort Zone' makes gym workout a pleasant routine, for anyone at any age and with a mobile body condition.

Workout routinely committed to on a regular basis, such as every-other-day, the 'comfort zone' will increase organically over time. It is exactly like the Chinese saying:
"Water becomes a river eventually" (水到渠成).

Figure 7.1
Ian Dowe during his World-Championship years

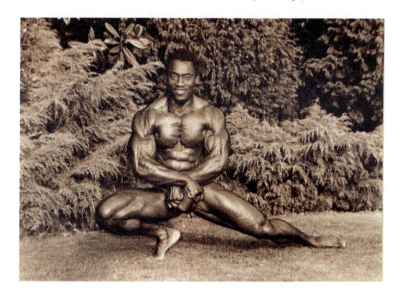

Source: Ian Dowe

Alternatively, adopting Dowe's Comfort Zone approach offers a shorter time to gain a result, considering that exertion in the gym can easily cause serious damage. In Asia, it is quite common to hear news of accidents in the gym because of this reason. Sometimes, too much weight beyond our capabilities can even cause death in certain cases.

In addition, Benjamin pointed out that "extreme exertion produces excess cortisol, (this is a stress hormone). Higher concentrations of cortisol breaks down muscle fibre and stores fat and you will achieve the **opposite result**". That's why I began to put weight on when I was in the Cycling Club at University.

Diet is as equally important as exercise. Before the first day in Dowe Dynamics Gym, I was asked by Ian to send him every single picture of what I ate. The reason was very simple, fully aligned with Chapter 4. Of course, what to eat directly becomes nutrition to the body, which directly converts to energy levels achieved in the gym. What to eat directly influences the outcome of a gym workout, in terms of how much you can achieve the muscle strength, body shape, and level of fitness.

Ian Dowe's top advice for fitness & muscle strength training includes:
- Only cooked from fresh: no processed food
- Balanced food: meat, vegetables, fish, a small amount of **carbohydrates**
- Solid food is preferred.
- No sugar: even fruits are allowed only occasionally
- Avoid eating out: bring your own meal when travelling
- Fresh/ organic vegetables

Ian Dowe's Comfort Zone methodology assisted me to stay fit and gain muscle strength easily, quickly, and maintained for a longer time. Because Ian requested my 100% perfect form/ posture compliance; he always took videos in every session (Figure 7.2).

Figure 7.2
On the 6th week training with Ian Dowe:
He always took video footage of my progress

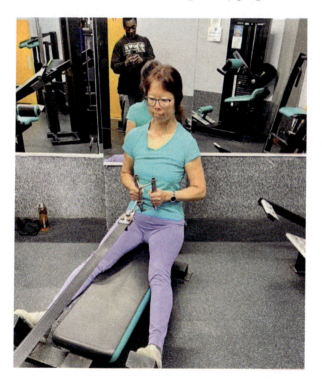

Source: Dr. I Han

Now I still do the workout every other day. If I travel, I find a local gym. If there is no gym, I can use other variations of weights or resistance bands. Gym workout has become what I never imagined before. Whenever I return to Dowe Dynamics Gym, I admire his numerous championship pictures on the walls (including Ian Dowe, Arnold Schwarzenegger, and many many well-known athletes and dancers) because I now understand the importance of excellence, persistence and commitment they applied to their gym ethic (Figure 7.3). If I cannot mould myself like them, (which was never my intention), I can become a woman with unimaginable strength in my 50s and beyond. I've become more confident in helping people with heavy luggage/baby strollers on stairs in the London Underground. I was able to carry more shopping bags (maybe you don't want to spend more money, so it is of no benefit to you). More importantly, whenever I have a pain in my lower back, (which has been an issue since my thirties), I am able to resolve it by lifting the right weights. Holding those weights pushes me back to my correct posture, which has been liberating for me.

Figure 7.3
Workout at the Gym Hall of Fame:
Dowe Dynamics Gym
London, UK

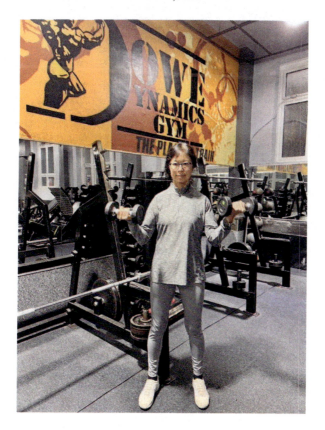

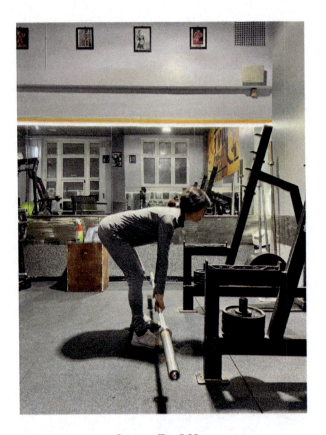

Source: Dr. I Han

When lifting the weights in the correct posture, it automatically corrects the "lazy posture" (Figure 7.4). Benjamin also confirmed my capability to hold my posture, even though I still need his treatment on my collapsed spine at times. But prior to the start of my weight training program, it was not easy to restore even after a fortnight's treatment. It has now become so simple to develop stronger muscle strength to hold my posture, better than ever before.

I then realised the simple beauty of Ian Dowe's 50+ years professional experience and his fundamental belief with his practice and process towards his impressive world championships as well as hundreds of students successfully trained by him.

The Comfort Zone methodology is simple and beautiful (it is a personal choice if you prefer a harder route, so be it).

Figure 7.4
Squat as the workout to correct my posture

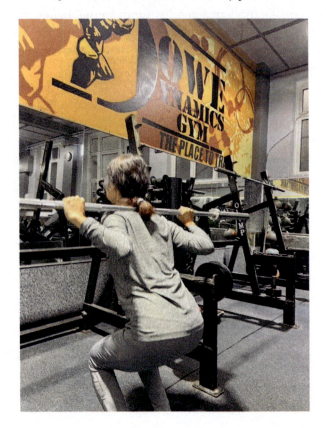

Source: Dr. I Han

Notes:

[1]
A friend, recently influenced by me, went to the gym to train her legs, concluding that the source of her knee pain from marathon running was connected to her weak legs.

[2]
My own discovery: Pai Da Gong (Chapter 6) four hours after workout makes the best recovery of muscle, Qi, and throughout the body.

Commentary

Benjamin Pluke

Founder of Benjamin Pluke Osteopathy
London, UK

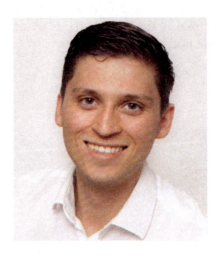

As a classical osteopath I examine the whole body of a patient, assessing how well it functions as an integrated system. Can the body stand, walk, squat and climb easily? Can the body remove waste, bring in nutrition through digestion, circulate efficiently, manage hormones and when relevant, manage the menstrual system?

I look at the overall structure of a body, how is the spine? Can it rest within a neutral posture while standing? Is the body able to climb and squat sufficiently?

While observing this, I assess the health of the skin, nails, hair, how someone is breathing, how much energy they have. Once the examination begins, it becomes clear how someone's digestive system, liver, menstrual organs, heart and lungs are functioning.

When I first met Dr Han, she was suffering from a lot of problems with her posture and digestion. This manifested in her neck, shoulder, mid back, lower back and hip. When I talk about neutral posture, I refer to the balance between a lordosis (the spine curving towards the front of the body) and a kyphosis (the spine curving away from the body). A neutral posture has one lordosis in the neck, one kyphosis in the mid back and one lordosis in the lower back. Any alteration from this in a standing posture, shows there is some form of mechanical inefficiency, which will either just reduce somebody's potential output across the board, or lead to a whole variety of unwanted symptoms. Dr Han unfortunately had kyphotic curves where there should be lordotic curves and lordotic curves where there should have been kyphotic curves. This was causing her symptoms, and putting tremendous strain on the rest of her health and well-being.

Before Dr Han started exercising with Ian Dowe, we had managed to recover her lordosis in her neck, and her kyphosis in her upper back. However, her lower back would frequently collapse back into a kyphosis, this was likely due to overall weakness in her muscular chain. After only a few weeks of following Ian Dowe's beginners methodology, her lower back posture had finally stabilised, her pelvis and rib cage, her shoulders and neck started developing more and more healthy movement. After continuing and completing eight weeks with Ian, the health that Dr Han had recovered was truly inspiring, she finally had achieved a stable neutral posture, with functional healthy muscle.

The exercises we choose to perform are also crucial, Ian Dowe's attention to detail with the technique used in the exercises and the arrangement of each workout, directly improves one's overall posture and mobility.

Another thing to consider is one of the most wonderful hormones in the body: Cortisol. It is spectacular in its role in keeping us alive, and getting us through the challenges of life. In healthy amounts at the right intervals in the day, it wakes us up in the morning, aids digestion of every meal and in general helps us think and move. However, it is categorised as a stress hormone, in higher concentrations it leads to muscle breakdown, fat storage, reduced immune activity and therefore reduced repair. Though there are many things that can contribute to this, over exercising, either during a training session (over exertion by lifting too heavy or for too long), or by not having adequate rest days or quality sleep. Another common issue people can struggle with, is due to the other demands of life, we become Cortisol deficient, we can burn through our supply and then normal function in the body is at best diminished. Therefore, not training to the point of failure is the best way to ensure consistent progress with exercise.

There are other health considerations, as our nutritional input is highly critical to our ability to stay healthy. There is a fungus called Candida Albicans which lives in our intestinal tract. One could say its role is to reduce initial blood sugar spiking from starch and carbohydrates in our food, by consuming it before our blood absorbs it. The downside to this, is that our modern, over processed diet has a huge amount of sugar in most meals and drinks, which leads to the candida having an overly favourable environment and our friendly flora in the microbiome less capacity to survive or space to thrive. The candida multiplies, and can inhabit the whole of the digestive tract, and then move through the blood to the rest of the body, hence leading to thrush as one example.

The other factor apart from sugar, that favours Candida and overall affects our ability to absorb nutrition is pH impact on the blood of the food we eat. When our body respires, and cells perform anaerobic or aerobic respiration, the waste material is acidic. If the blood moves out of a narrow band of pH, we will become very unwell and eventually die. Therefore, there are systems in the body that buffer the acidity in the blood, to keep us healthy, our lungs, liver and kidneys, to keep it simple. If our food or meal leans towards an acidic pH, our liver will prioritise keeping us alive rather than assisting in digestion. This leads to general swelling in the body, due to inadequately digested food creating unwanted chemicals which stress our immune system. Additionally, the acidic environment in the intestines favours the Candida and harms our own microbiome.

However, this impact is relatively simple to negate, we need to balance the pH of our meals, most vegetables are alkaline when digested and animal fats and proteins are acidic. Therefore, eat vegetables with meat and animal products. Carbohydrates in wheat and potatoes are also greatly overlooked, and these essentially digest as sugar, the pizza and pasta meals, are incredibly high in sugar, which leads to overall stress on our organs.

Commentary

Ian Dowe

Mr. Universe, IFBB World Championships

Founder of Dowe Dynamics Gym
London, UK

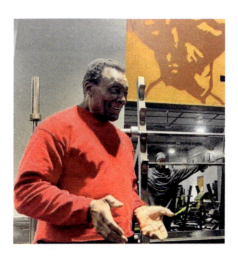

Dr. Han was probably one of my best students because of her commitment. She made significant progress in the first two weeks while other people might spend several months or years to achieve. She paid attention to the food/ diet which is very important to train and get a result.

However, everyone is different. Just be yourself. Do what you can do. Sometimes you are stronger and sometimes you are weaker. If you feel stronger, lift more weights. If you feel weaker, reduce the weight. That's really simple!

There are many training styles, just like many different schools of Chinese Martial Arts. I trained myself to achieve multiple British, European, and World Championships. Also, I trained many other Champions. So, my bespoke training philosophy works. No matter which style of training you choose, you have to make sure it will work for you.

Currently more and more middle-aged clients come to me to ask for training to increase muscle strength. My method is really simple: find a routine according to your level of fitness, and get a result. It is very personal. Never compare yourself with other people. But, there is a universal formula: exercise, eat, and rest.

Chapter 8

Implications & Getting Started

I am so grateful that I've received so much guidance to achieve this level of health. Ultimately for myself I consider it an amazing achievement:

Freedom.

I lost the excess weight that does not belong to my body. I achieved muscle strength by easy exercise and training. All these made me feel more freedom to enjoy life.

I can wear a beautiful dress which in the past held no interest for me.
I can offer to carry luggage or strollers for others with full confidence.
I can eat when I want to eat, or I don't have to eat if there is nothing good to eat.
I can stay in a cheap but excellent accommodation in the city centre, eventhough it is nine floors of stairs to climb from the ground.

Weight loss and muscle strength, simply, lead you take more control of your life, and you will enjoy freedom of life (Figure 8.1). I can jump as high as I did when I was dancing in primary school (without damaging myself at the age over 50).

Figure 8.1
Freedom of life

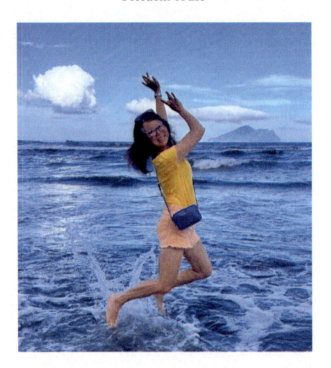

Source: Dr. I Han

1. **Freedom to eat:**
   Choose what to eat, when to eat, whether you would like to eat in a restaurant or at home. It's your choice.

2. **Freedom to exercise:**
   Whether walking, cycling, jogging, or going to a gym does not make it painful at all, and those exercises will not damage your body because of

your muscle strength. If you like running, train your legs more, and then you will not suffer from knee or ankle pains.

3. **Freedom to move:**
   Whether a budget economy class or a luxury business class, you enjoy more space and, also, you don't mind the in-flight food at all (because you don't have to eat it if you don't like it). When travelling, you can walk more, shop more, and take more beautiful pictures (maybe climb up to the top).

4. **Freedom to share:**
   Whether you would like to share your ultimate experience on social media, to help more people, or to share your knowhow as a business, they all create more positive energy.

By reading this book, you might already get an idea that it is not difficult at all to start your own journey and move towards your own **Freedom.**

Find your Comfort Zone to get started.

Your Comfort Zone will make sure that you will not dislike what you are going to do. It will also eventually build into your routine and become your lifestyle.

Figure 8.2
Holistic view: Long-term lifestyle

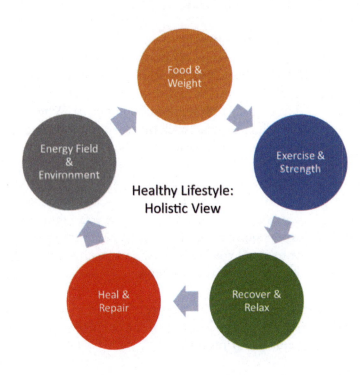

Source: Dr. I Han

Ready to get started?

When you take an action on losing the weight and on building muscle strength, it is the goal to achieve a holistic view of a healthy lifestyle (Figure 8.2):

1. **Food & Weight (orange)**: According to Chapter 4, you can start with the guidelines of right/good food to eat (Table 4.1) and re-adjust yourself according to your own body conditions throughout the time. Follow the true feelings of your body, do not follow your "head". Eventually, you can create your own guidelines of what you enjoy eating most of the time. It might be different from my Table 4.1. You will gradually go "back" to your right body weight, in a balanced state.

2. **Exercise & Strength (blue)**: According to Chapter 6, maybe start with the easiest Pai Da Gong exercise if you haven't got one comfortable routine yet. Or, maybe you enjoy Yoga or another less demanding exercise. Spend 30-60 minutes on an easy exercise every day or at least every other day. Gradually, the routine exercise will help to create muscle strength or increase muscle resistance. If you already go to the gym, make sure the exercise is what you really "enjoy" throughout the time. If you've got a trainer, make sure he/ she understands what will only benefit your muscle strength, but not damage you at all.

3. **Recover & Relax (green)**: As a lifestyle, it has to be consistent in the long run. Therefore, either diet or exercise, sometimes you have to relax, and sometimes, it takes time to recover if you've done too much that causes uncomfortable feelings (including eating too much).

4. **Heal & Repair (red)**: To find what suits you, it is a trial-and-error process. You have to re-examine, re-adjust, and re-adapt according to your own condition on the day-to-day basis. If you cause damage to yourself, do not continue your routine. Stop to heal and get some trustworthy expert to repair you before you re-start. The worst case is always to expand the damage when you already have an injury.

5. **Energy field & Environment (grey)**: According to Chapter 5, a holistic view starts from our own "small universe" and involves/ interacts with our surrounding environment as many levels of the "larger universe". There are many books that keep telling us: positive energy creates a good energy field, or your good wish will come true (*e.g.*, Rhonda Byrne's *The Secret*, Eckhart Tolle's *The Power of Now*, …), which will be discussed further in Chapter 9.

The holistic view of a long-term lifestyle shift, you can start from any one of the above five. Just pick whatever colour(s) you think it is easy to start with, and grow the circle from there. For example, I started from **Food & Weight**, without exercise. After I lost most of the weight that did not belong to me, I then started **Exercise & Strength**, firstly, Pai Da Gong, and secondly, gym workout. A new finding after I started to be trained in the gym: doing Pai Da Gong four hours after gym workout is very effective to relax the tight muscles and restore the Qi throughout meridian pathways. Comfort Zone gym training plus Pai Da Gong causes no pain for me.

The common thought in the gym "no pain, no gain" becomes "no pain, only gain".

Relaxation after any exercise is extremely important. Pai Da Gong is highly recommended to try, if you do not have a good method of relaxation after exercise.

Sometimes, however, it might take more time to **Recover & Relax** after exercises if my body condition is not in balance. Sometimes, I have to go to healers to treat my pain from over-exercise or wrong posture (still happens if I am not careful enough). When I went to other gyms during the travel, I could not believe how many people conducted workout in the wrong way, which I should have told them to stop if I were their trainer. It is regrettable that I was not able to tell them, but instead looked at what they've done to damage their structures. In the future, I am committed to launching an education programme by communicating the importance of how the right exercise helps, but wrong exercise hurts.

Finally, when I improved my body to a healthier and stronger state (less waste in my body and less energy spent on holding weak muscles), I could feel how the **Energy Field & Environment** have an impact on me. Thus, I can arrange more time to be close to the natural environment without artificial disturbances and get a true **Heal & Repair** by being away from negative impact created by artificial disturbances. Figure 8.2 is an integrative system, with arrows as I experienced, and without arrows if you would like to start all of them simultaneously.

The methodology you might consider, could be more "scientific" by controlling other variables while experimenting one major variable you care for the most at a time. Take **Food & Weight** as an example, Figure 8.3 demonstrates one method for your own research, according to what is illustrated in Figure 5.1 regarding the laboratory test principle. Even though the human body is an extremely complicated system as a whole, where most internal and external variables change all the time, we can still follow the principle to approximately find out what is right or not.

So, if you would like to find out whether wheat-based food like bread (01) influences your weight, you might start to completely stop the wheat in your diet for a while (give yourself a time, say, at least two weeks). During the period of your research, eat rice or other gluten-free carbohydrates (05), while keeping all other food unchanged (within your daily routine selections) as usual (02, 03, 04). After that, you will see the result from your own experiment. This method can further extend to any food/ diet and exercise that you suspect might not be right for you.

Do your own research, because only you know yourself what's the best. As long as you know what you are doing, and make sure there is no harm, by working within your Comfort Zone, everything is worth trying, one at a time.

Figure 8.3
Methodology: Your Own Research

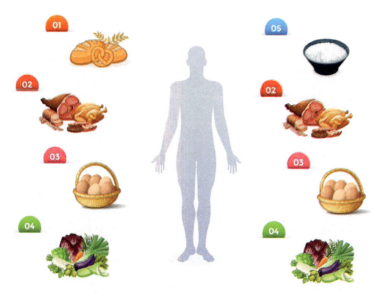

Source: Livy Sung

Finally, it is the time to take action.

Table 8.1 is a template for you to formulate an action plan for your own experiment. Each time, experiment only one major variable on the left blue column during at least a 2-week window, while keeping all other routine as usual. Start from a food/ diet variable, and also create another table by applying exercise variables when you are ready to exercise.

Table 8.1
Action Plan:
your own experiment

Food/ Diet variable	Choices	Check points
Stable saturated fat to heat/cook with	<ul><li>Animal fat (duck, chicken, pork…)</li><li>Coconut oil</li><li>Ghee</li></ul>	☐ Lose/gain weight Feel healthy / ill ☐ Get more / less energy ☐ Some illness / pain: reduced / increased ☐ Nothing changed
No unnecessary sugar	<ul><li>No sugar additives at all</li><li>Small amount of low-sugar fruits (*e.g.* berries)</li></ul>	☐ Very difficult (additive to sugar)/not difficult ☐ Lose / gain the weight ☐ Feel healthy / ill ☐ Get more / less energy ☐ Some illness / pain: reduced / increased ☐ Nothing changed
A. Fermented food & drink with meals	<ul><li>Kimchi</li><li>Miso</li><li>Kombucha</li><li>Yogurt</li><li>Kefir</li><li>Cheese</li></ul>	☐ Digestion improved / constipation ☐ Lose / gain weight ☐ Feel healthy / ill ☐ Get more/less energy ☐ Some illness / pain: reduced / increased

(raw / unpasteurised)		☐ Nothing changed
Carbohydrates in the last meal	▪ Protein, fat, vegetables in earlier meal(s)	☐ Lose / gain weight ☐ Get more / less energy during the day ☐ Less/ easy to get hungry ☐ Nothing changed
B. Eat only when you are hungry (not your head to tell you it is the time to be hungry)	▪ No other snacks/ food between major meals ▪ Reduce to two meals a day (no over-eating, but feel satisfied)	☐ Digestion improved / constipation ☐ Lose/ gain the weight ☐ Feel healthy / ill ☐ Get more / less energy ☐ Some illness/ pain: reduced / increased ☐ Nothing changed
C. (you name it) …………..		
D. (many more in further details) …………..		

Source: Dr. I Han

Similarly, you can create another table for your exercise experiment. For example, if you have been running for a while, but started to feel knee pain, you might add a relaxation session after your running, such as Pai Da Gong or stretch for at least 30 minutes afterwards. If it is not helping after two weeks, you might consider training your legs with a professional trainer and then return to running.

After you set up your own Table 8.1, I propose three strategies for yourself:

lazy, ambitious, and balanced.

The difference between these three is how you get started and make progress within your Comfort Zone. Please remember:
Comfort Zone is defined (in this book): within your own limits and feeling comfortable, without stress. It is a dynamic concept. It does not mean anything negatively.

In the short term, your Comfort Zone moves up and down according to your physical and mental conditions. In the long term, your comfort zone evolves and eventually shifts to the next level. As shown in Figure 8.4:

- **Lazy Strategy**: enjoy the bottom or close to the bottom of your Comfort Zone. Keep it easy but you still make progress over time. This is closer to my own strategy. If you think you are a lazy person like me, this is probably an easy way to get started. It's much better than never getting started!

- **Ambitious Strategy**: push to the limit or close to the top of your Comfort Zone. Do your best, but do not push yourself into a painful or stressful place. Make sure you always enjoy what you do.

- **Balance Strategy**: stay with what you are comfortable to do. Feel a little extra space that you might be able to work harder if you really want to, but probably not all the time.

The level of your Comfort Zone includes the physical and mental state of you when you eat, exercise and rest, holistically within your specific environment. For example, when you've been buried in a project before deadlines, you want to eat more but it feels hard to lift the weights you normally can. Thus, you could eat three or four times a day (while you normally eat two meals a day), and maybe a delicious dessert in the afternoon tea-time (while you normally do not have a dessert with your afternoon tea), if it provides you a moment of relaxation. When you travel, it might not be easy to find a gym or a time to stick to your daily routine. Then you can reduce the frequency or the strength of your exercise, and give yourself more time to relax and have fun.

Up and down, everyone has good and bad times or conditions.

Stay in your Comfort Zone, as always, you can still make progress in the long run.

More importantly, you will keep on your track upwards, which is much better than feeling it's too hard to keep on track and give up.

Why bother with a short time of ups and downs?

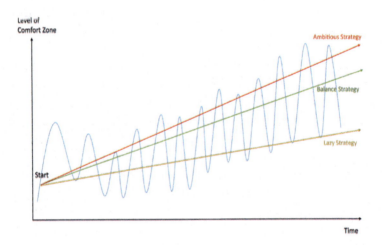

Figure 8.4
Find Your Comfort Zone:
Lazy, Balance, or Ambitious Strategy

Source: Dr. I Han

Table 8.2 is a guide for you to get started and progress over time, within your Comfort Zone. Take an action following one of the three strategies. For most people, as human nature, I recommend starting with the Lazy Strategy. Once you find out it is easy to achieve, you might want to switch to Balance Strategy. Sometimes, you may probably demand a faster result and Ambitious Strategy is a fast track without spending the extra time.

It is only up to you to make a choice of how fast / how easy, within your Comfort Zone you would like to get a result. Holistically, slow track or fast track, it will eventually become a healthy lifestyle in the long term. You will enjoy the freedom because you can easily manage a right weight and muscle strength.

Table 8.2
Strategies towards a holistic view of a healthy lifestyle

Strategy	Style	Action	Check List
Lazy	bottom of your Comfort Zone	• Food/Diet: Avoid the wrong food/ingredients, and eat happily. • Exercise: Do an easy exercise at least every other day for at least 30 minutes.	☐ If it becomes too easy, eat 10% less and/or eat close to 100% right. ☐ If it is too easy, increase the duration and/or frequency of exercise.
Ambitious	push to the limit of your Comfort Zone	• Food/Diet: Stick only to the right food/ingredients. • Exercise: Do a serious exercise that you	☐ If it becomes easy, eat only one meal a day with the same amount per meal if you do not feel hungry. ☐ If it becomes easy to manage,

133

		can manage without pain, every other day for at least 30 minutes.	increase the intensity / duration frequency of the exercise.
Balance	Up & down within your Comfort Zone	<ul><li>Food/ Diet</li><li>Exercise</li></ul>In between Lazy and Ambitious strategies, depending on whether you have time to cook / exercise, or whether you are happy to do more or not.	☐ Up & down is very normal, so is this strategy-- sometimes you want to achieve more in a short period of time, sometimes you don't.

Source: Dr. I Han

Once you put yourself in the process, the process will carry you through. I shared my journey with you, now it is your turn.

Remember the movie "Minority Report"?
Don't trust anyone, including me.

Do your own research.
Experiment yourself.

Weight and muscle always tell the truth about your body, as an everyday message whenever you walk, run, lift, or even just sit or stand still.

Find your Comfort Zone and stay in it, so it can sustain itself easily.

Comfort Zone will develop itself gradually.

Everything is possible!

What else should I teach?

This is it.

Chapter 9

Qi-Gong Healer, Quantum, and Beyond

Nothing is impossible.

In the quantum world, everything is possible.

Academic research all ends at "limitation" and "future research". This chapter is not the ending chapter, but the one that opens to the "future research" along this journey. Meanwhile, there is no limitation because of the infinite universe.

"The start determines the end", 以始為終 in Chinese. It means:
The start leads to the end, and the end leads to the start.
It is exactly in line with the Yin-Yang philosophy in the I Ching (易經).

It is not an analogy, but a fact of my personal journey shared in all previous chapters. At the end of the book, I would like to discuss the "official start" of this journey with a senior Qi-Gong healer, Mr. Han-Ching Lin, whom I met in Taichung in 2015. Mr. Lin only received his primary school diploma, yet displays more wisdom and scientific knowledge than many people with university degrees. Similar to my experience with the many farmers I met, what I've learned from Mr. Lin until the day I moved to England, was certainly an invaluable life-and mind changing experience.

I visited Mr. Lin to be treated by his Qi-Gong every Monday afternoon during 2015-2019. I did not have any significant illness to be "treated" because I wanted to discover how good he was in order to save my father's life from the outset. My father sadly died in his 80's in the Venetian Hospital Taipei later in 2016. While my father was not lucky to have Mr. Lin treating him, I did.

Upon reflection it finally occurred to me after my first lengthy session with Mr Lin that I, like my father, was heading for a potential heart attack. Mr Lin guided me to realise that my heart area was always bruised for almost an entire week after each of Mr. Lin's treatment. This is a sign of a potential heart attack risk because of Qi- and/or blood-blockage. That also explained my earlier inquest why I was completely dizzy and could not stand at all, one day after the end of a class I taught in the University before 2015. The department officer called an ambulance to send me to a hospital where the doctors spent four hours checking my heart and many other conditions, but nothing was discovered or resolved.

During those five years of regular treatment with Mr. Lin, I enjoyed every conversation during my three+ hours there. He shared many "stories" behind the *I Ching*, Feng Shui, Qi Gong, and much more. To me, as an academic researcher, by using the field-study method, I do not judge the information I receive, but only keep it. Later on, I might get a chance to verify the validation of the previous information from other sources or evidence. I then returned to tell Mr.

Lin what he said before I discovered would be real. Throughout these years, I then built up my own theory beyond academic narratives (like many yellows in Figure 1.1). By comparing my profession in academia, I gradually understood the gap between ancient wisdom and modern science.

What is Qi?

When I asked many western friends who have been practising Qi-Gong for years or decades, they only knew the term as a "name" of those movements.

Qi is 氣 in Mandarin. Originally the Chinese character symbolised steam above rice. This signifies the intangible and elusive nature of Qi. If you about know Chinese medicine, you know that Qi is the vital circulation around the body, in addition to blood circulation, to keep the human body fully functioning and alive.

Imagine a balloon, or Qi-Chui (氣球) in mandarin. The Kung-Qi (空氣, air, or empty space full of Qi, while Kung means space/ empty) inside the balloon supporting its shape, as either round, heart, or even a mickey mouse shape. When the Qi reduces over days, some part of the balloon deflates sooner and other parts deflate later. I found this an easy analogy to understand the Qi inside a human body. Western science cannot see or measure Qi, as it has a quality of "emptiness" and intangibility, just like the air (Kung-Qi) inside a balloon. If Qi moves smoothly, the physical human body can be supported, just like the perfection of a balloon as it is designed to be. If Qi is blocked somewhere, the physical human body seeks to be biased and supported, just like a balloon loses its air gradually. In the beginning, the person might only feel not so well, maybe just a lack of energy or a headache, perhaps breathing harder than usual. When a person attends a Western hospital, doctors and machines might all report normal readings (like my earlier case of dizziness). My own incident might have been because the Qi was completely blocked by all other channels [1] to a specific organ in the body, just like a balloon going down completely.

Outside the body, there is Qi from the ground/earth, Qi from the air/space, and the universe. The harmony between "small universe" and "big universe" is the simple yet fundamental theory to support physical health, mental health, and further develop spiritual advancement on this planet within the infinite universe.

In addition to Mr. Lin, later I met a few more Qi Gong healers/ masters in Taiwan. Ms. Liu is a Feng-shui master based in Taoism. Another, Mr. Lin Kun-Lo in Taipei, who has been famous for Shaolin Qi-Gong healing, started to treat me and my mum during my holiday in Taipei. As I was an old friend of one of Mr. Lin's previous Qi-Gong students, there was an immediate connection and trust between us. He shared a lot of insights during a very short period of time when I was there. On my last trip I went to receive treatment with two other British people who had practised Qi-Gong for many years. They were amazed how effective the treatment could re-generate the Qi inside the body and get healed. There are numerous masters in Taiwan and maybe other parts of the world. I invite you to open your mind and explore it for yourself. As you make a wish, the infinite universe will present some golden offers to you.

I studied physics for two years at the National Taiwan University. Quantum energy is understood but there is so much more beyond what we understand, the Physics researcher had explained to us. Many of my previous physics classmates started to study Chinese medicine, Qi-Gong, and religions while they discovered the limitations of modern sciences. If you don't agree with ancient Chinese wisdom, there are many other western studies such as Lester and Parker's book *"What Really Makes You Ill?"* worth reading to get different perspectives.

Beyond the academic head, the heart, Qi, energy, and the harmony among the universe is the key to open your future.

Weight loss and muscle strength, this book ends here with the start of a journey for you and me. Comfort Zone strategies towards freedom are not only for you, but for all of us in this infinite universe.

I offer my love from my angels and masters to all of you.

Good luck!

Note:
[1]
There are many channels of Qi circulating inside the body, the same as blood. If a small blockage happens in the circulatory system, the blood will detour to support the organ via other channels until they are all blocked.

Commentary

Mr. Lin, Han-Ching

40 years as a Qi Gong Healer
Taichung, Taiwan

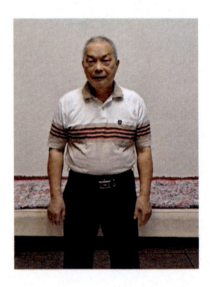

I Ching, Feng-Shui, Bagua (易經風水八卦) all told the same thing:
the operation of the universe, and they have been there to guide for thousands of years.

Yin leads Yang, Yang leads Lin, Yin and Yang give birth to all and are endless. It is believed that a short nap in heaven roughly equals 20 years on this planet. Everyone on earth was sent to experience here, or a human life, as a journey.

Everyone has his/her mission in this life. The universe arranges what to happen and what not to. If you are a good person, the universe will always give you a hand. If the environment/field/person is right for you, you stay; otherwise, you leave.

I've been a Qi Gong healer for decades. Who comes and who leaves, I am aware.

But I will not tell until the moment it appears. It also depends on the consciousness level of each person. It takes time or lives to get to a point when you realise what you are doing and why you are here.

Qi Gong healing is simple as it explains itself as healing by using Qi Gong, or Qi as an energy source.

Where there is a blockage inside a body, there is the illness. I heal the patients by using my healing-Qi to clear the blockage. It takes time to heal, and it takes time to recover. How well the body can incorporate Qi-energy depends on how long, after the treatment, the body can stay in the unblocked or balanced state. Daily life in the modern world might create a challenge for us to keep in a balanced state, or an energy equilibrium, both physically and mentally.

The universe is naturally arranged. If you enjoy life with an easy mind, it will not be so difficult to find your balanced state, being in harmony with the universe.

Commentary

Seyhan Riza

20 years researcher & practitioner in the ways of natural healing & longevity
London, UK

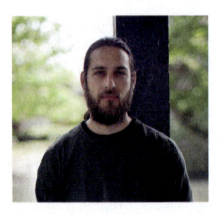

From early in my life, I spent most of my younger years living between two worlds, that of village life out on a small island surrounded by nature and that of city life of London. This unbeknownst to me would give me an experiential knowledge of how these two ways of life can have an effect on our physical and mental health. From this I spent most of my teenage years experimenting with the effects of this type of duality up until my early twenties, which is when I immersed myself fully in research of natural modality's that have existed from ancient antiquity up to the present age by rediscovering what has been passed down to us through time immemorial. Since that time, I have been studying and practising the systems of Chinese herbal medicine,

Ayurveda (Indian medical system), Dry Fasting, Agriculture/soil culture, Biochemistry, Biology, Bio Geometry, Epigenetics, Solar Terrestrial Physics, and Sound/ Frequency Healing.

When I first met Dr Han two and half years ago, given my background, I was very interested in what she was doing in Taiwan and the people she was meeting with. We had a few conversations and I could see then that she was very adept at wanting to push through what she had learned, being academically trained for most part of her life and explore a deeper meaning of what the world had to offer. Since that time, I have seen her grow and adapt not only her mental awareness, but also the physical along with her spirituality in leaps and bounds.

Changing her diet and lifestyle routines allowed her to lose weight and become more physically fit and healthy, which in turn then saw a marked increase in her focus and mental determination. After these changes her quest for comprehending the totality of these combined experiences I feel has brought her spiritually to a place where now she can look on her future with a more holistic view and her manifesting abilities are to me proof of the deeper connection she is forming within herself and to the world around her.

Now having had the chance to travel to Taiwan and meet some of these amazing people, getting my own direct experience with two well renowned Qi Gong healers, was an experience that has profoundly affected me and will carry with me for the rest of my life. Both times just being in the presence of these amazing healers gave me a sense and feeling of great honour and that buzz of energy that only few can produce and that was before having any treatment. During and after both treatments I can only say that the experience of having my own body's energy manipulated in such fashions left me with a deeper understanding of not only within myself but of how these connections can be used to create balance internally and then out to the world around us, and a high that was immediate and lasted for days afterwards.

Along with 20+ years of practice and personal experience in this field, I begin to see the bigger picture in how Qi/energy is really the foundation to how our mental and physical bodies function to maintain balance in both internal and external worlds. Knowing this it is clear to me that since energy is the fundamental building blocks to creation itself, this is where healing begins and in fact all living begins.

As even now mainstream science is starting to catch up with the age-old notion that everything is energy, the study of Quantum is now becoming the leading field to explore, in order to understand the connection between the all (macrocosm / microcosm). As above so below as stated by Thoth (high priest of ancient Egypt). So given this, it is easy to see why the energy that everything is made of, including ourselves, is the very thing that connects us all.

References

Avena, NM, Rada, P, Hoebel, BG. 2008. Evidence for sugar addiction: behavioral and neurochemical effects of intermittent, excessive sugar intake. *Neuroscience & Biobehavioral Reviews*, 32 (1): 20-39.

Davis, William. 2021. *Wheat Belly Total Health*. HarperCollins Publisher: London.

Dunning, August. 2020. *The Phoenix Protocol Dry Fasting for Rapid Healing and Radical Life Extension: Functional Immortality*.

Lester, Dawn & Parker, David. 2019. *What Really Makes You Ill?* Amazon: UK.

Han, I & Hou, Sheng-tsung. 2016. *Social Innovation and Business in Taiwan*. Palgrave Macmillan: New York, USA.

Huang, Li-Chun. 2011. *Auricular Diagnosis: Procedures, Directions, and Methods*. Auricular Medicine Center: Alabama, USA.

Mitleton-Keely, Eve, Paraskevas, Alexandros, and Day, Christopher. 2018. *Handbook of Research Methods in Complexity Science: Theory and Practice* (eds). Edward Elgar Publishing: Glos, UK.

Sheldrake, Rupert. 2012. *The Science Delusion*. Hodder & Stoughton Ltd: London, UK.

Tyler, Sheena E.B. 2017. Nature's electric potential: A systematic review of the role of bioelectricity in wound healing and regenerative processes in animals, humans, and plants. *Frontiers in Physiology*, Vol. 8, Article 627.

Yang, Jwing-ming. 1992. *Chinese Qigong Massage: General Message*. Yang's Martial Arts Association (YMAA): MA, USA.

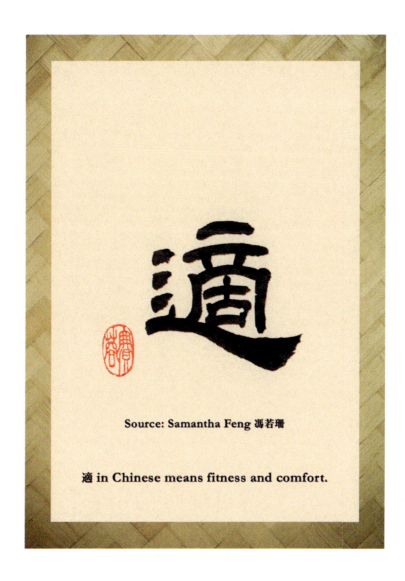

Source: Samantha Feng 馮若珊

適 in Chinese means fitness and comfort.

Printed in Great Britain
by Amazon